EXPERTS AGREE: THIS TRANSFORMATIONAL BOOK IS A LANDMARK ON THE PATH TO JOYFUL, GUILT-FREE LIVING

"The first great therapy book of the Nineties . . . a book I highly recommend to all."

—Brian L. Weiss, M.D.
Chairman, Department of Psychiatry
Mount Sinai Medical Center, Florida, and
author of *Many Lives, Many Masters*

"The gifted healer has revealed her nature as a gifted teacher! I had expected to like the book, but I hadn't expected to be transformed by it. This is a book to which others that follow will be compared as a standard."

—Steven E. Locke, M.D.
Director, Medical Student Education
Assistant Professor of Psychiatry, Harvard Medical School, and
co-author of *The Healer Within*

"A simple and convincing course towards peace of mind and heart. Dr. Borysenko paints with great artistry the details of the anvil of guilt upon which so many of us hammer ourselves."

—Jon Kabat-Zinn, Ph.D.
Director, the Stress Reduction Clinic,
University of Massachusetts Medical Center, and
author of *Full Catastrophe Living*

"An intricate tapestry of personal experiences, moving insights, latest scientific discoveries, and genuine, deeply felt spiritual wisdom. . . . An exquisite and emotional landmark of a book."

—Dr. Kenneth Pelletier
Associate Clinical Professor of Medicine,
University of California, and
author of *Mind as Healer, Mind as Slayer*

"Profound and delightfully readable . . . a major contribution to the literature on healing the person and healing the planet."

—**Willis Harman**
President, The Institute of Noetic Sciences

"The book is wise and gentle, and at the same time strong and clear. Joan's insights . . . are truly transformative."

—**Jeremy Taylor**
author of *Dream Work*

"An engaging, insightful distillation of psychological and spiritual wisdom and healing."

—*Kirkus Reviews*

"A marvelous, powerful, and important book."

—**Barbara Dossey, R.N., M.S.**
co-author of *Holistic Nursing: A Handbook for Practice*

"I applaud her. . . . We are, as spiritual seekers and new age physicians, recognizing holiness in the whole human person, and Joan is on the cutting edge in acknowledging these discoveries."

—**Reverend Barbara Fitterer,**
Saint Andrews Ross, California

"A manual for self-healing, a guide book for exploring the wounds of childhood and using that confrontation as a vehicle for spiritual growth. It's a marvelous blend of the psychological and the transcendent, an antidote to malaise."

—**Daniel Goleman,**
author of *The Meditative Mind*

"A groundbreaking work in the understanding of the relationship of guilt, love and the Source of Life—God. Our eyes are opened to the possibilities of healing not available to us before."

—**Reverend John J. Malecki,**
head of the Consultation Center in Albany

"Well-researched . . . it offers excellent meditation ideas that will help the reader come on through the guilt to the love."

—**Jack D. Kern**
Minister of the Unity of Naples Church, Naples, Florida

"A wise and wonderful book . . . a book of enormous help. . . . Joan is not afraid to question the conventional wisdoms, and what impressed me most is that she questions the so-called New Age conventional wisdoms along with the old."

—**James A. Autry**
President of the Magazine Group and author of *Life after Mississippi*

JOAN BORYSENKO, PH.D., has been called "a rare jewel: respected scientist, gifted therapist, and unabashed mystic."* In 1987, she published the *New York Times* bestseller *Minding the Body, Mending the Mind*, the landmark work that helped thousands of medical patients to enhance their physical health by using the power of the mind. The co-founder and former director of the Mind/Body Clinic, New England Deaconess Hospital, Dr. Borysenko has established herself worldwide as a cellular biologist, a psychotherapist, an instructor of meditation, and a pioneer of the fascinating medical synthesis known as psychoimmunology. She is founder and president of Mind/Body Health Sciences, a consulting company to individuals, businesses, and hospitals.

*Dean Ornish, M.D.

GUILT IS THE TEACHER, LOVE IS THE LESSON

by Joan Borysenko, Ph.D.

A Time Warner Company

Grateful acknowledgment is made to the following for permission to reprint from:

The Kabir Book by Robert Bly. Copyright © 1971, 1977 by Robert Bly. Copyright © 1977 by The Seventies Press. Reprinted by permission of Beacon Press.

The Prophet by Kahlil Gibran by permission of Alfred Knopf, Inc. Copyright © 1923 by Kahlil Gibran, renewed 1951 by Administrators C.T.A. of Kahlil Gibran Estate and Mary G. Gibran.

Being Peace by Thich Nhat Hanh. Copyright © 1987 by Thich Nhat Hanh. Reprinted by permission of Parallax Press.

Thomas Merton: *Collected Poems of Thomas Merton*. Copyright © 1962, 1968 by the Abbey of Gethsemani. Reprinted by permission of New Directions Publishing Corporation. U.S. and Canadian rights; for British rights, refer to:

Gerald Pollinger Esq.
Laurence Pollinger
18 Maddox Street
Mayfair, London W1R OEU
ENGLAND

Emmanuel's Book: A Manual for Living Comfortably in the Cosmos by Pat Rodegast. Copyright © 1985 by Pat Rodegast. Reprinted by permission of Bantam Books.

Warner Books, Inc., 1271 Avenue of the Americas, New York, NY 10020
A Time Warner Company

Printed in the United States of America
First Trade Printing: May 1991
10 9 8 7

Library of Congress Cataloging-in-Publication Data

Borysenko, Joan.
Guilt is the teacher, love is the lesson / Joan Borysenko.
p. cm.
Includes bibliographical references.
ISBN 0-446-39224-3
1. Spiritual life. 2. Healing. 3. New Age movement. 4. Health.
I. Title.
BL624.B62 1990
152.4—dc20 89-27834
CIP

Designed by Giorgetta Bell McRee
Cover designed by Karen Katz
Photo by Sara McVicker

To the memory and living presence
of my parents,

Edward Zakon

and

Lillian Rubenstein Zakon

Nothing is precious
except that part of you which is in other people
and that part of others which is in you.
Up there
on high,
everything is one.

—Pierre Teilhard de Chardin
version by Blanche Gallagher

ACKNOWLEDGMENTS

This book is precious to me because it is about the stories of our lives, the way we are teachers and supporters of each other. I am grateful to all the people who have guided me along the way, to those who have shared joys and sorrows, and to those who have allowed me to be a guide in their physical, emotional, and spiritual healing. Through these interactions I have also found healing. May our ongoing stories, our struggles, and our victories be a shared framework and support as we learn to use our love and enthusiasm to bring into being a world of compassion.

A special thanks to my friends and former colleagues at the New England Deaconess Hospital whose bright minds and warm hearts contributed so much both to this book and to me. Thanks to the Mind/Body crew—my family away from home for many years—Steve Maurer, Olivia Hoblitzelle, and Jane Alter. Thanks to Eileen Stuart, Malini Ennis, Jane Leserman, Leo Stolbach, Ursula Brandt, and Herbert Benson, who created a unique environment for learning and growth. Thanks also to Rachel Naomi Remen, Robin Casarjian, Catherine Morrison, Steven Locke, Tom Stewart, Ilan Kutz, Harriett Mann, David Eisenberg, Jon Kabat-Zinn, David McClelland, and Gail Price, other colleagues whose ideas, insights, and support I gratefully acknowledge. I particularly want to thank Maureen Whalen for her careful search of the psychological literature on guilt for this book.

Because the ideas in this book are as old as antiquity and come from such a richness of sources, I have not always been able to remember where or from whom I first heard them. My apologies and thanks to anyone whose work may not have been explicitly credited.

To Indra's net, those shining spirits who were there to catch me in the soul's dark night: Steve Maurer, Olivia Hoblitzelle, Rachel Naomi Remen, Robin Casarjian, Harriett Mann, Beverly Feinberg-Moss, my brother, Alan, and my husband, Myrin. Thank you for holding me in my pain, and for guiding my safe passage through the rebirth canal! To Rick Ingrasci and Peggy Taylor, thanks for Hollyhock and Wellspring, for reviewing the manuscript, and especially for your friendship and love, which have meant so much to Myrin and me. Thanks also to Celia Hubbard, a.k.a. "Mother Goose," for the rich supply of love, inspiration, photographs, books, and ideas.

Natalia, Justin, and Andrei, dear children, what a lot we've learned together already. Your support in my work, in reminding me to play, and, most of all, your love means everything to me. Thanks, guys. And Myrin, beloved partner, soulmate, playmate, colleague, and best friend, thank you for your ever-deepening love and the tireless support that has helped manifest our vision.

To Mom and Dad, there's so much to say that I must depend upon your hearts to read between the lines here. Your love and care have meant so much to me, as have all the passages we moved through together. Growing up, growing old, fighting and learning, hurts and healings, births and deaths. I wish you had lived to see your grandchildren growing up, Dad—to see me growing up, for that matter. But we know you are there. And, Mom, even though you had hoped to live until this book was published, the courage you showed in facing both life and death are here in its pages. Thanks for your patience and your love. God bless you both.

And to Helen Rees, friend and literary agent extraordinaire, thanks for your faith in me and for making this all possible. To Bob Aylmer, at Lifecycle Learning, thanks for sponsoring the national workshop tour that helped hone some of these insights and practical processes for healing guilt. And, finally, I am most grateful to my patient and skillful editor at Warner Books, Joann Davis, whose encouragement and insight through many drafts has enriched this book tremendously.

CONTENTS

A Personal Introduction to Guilt and Healing 1

PART ONE/*Psychological Beginnings* 7

CHAPTER ONE/*Bodymind and Soul: A Psychospiritual Perspective on Guilt* 9

The Bodymind 10
Soul and Spirit—Individual Consciousness or One Mind? 14
Spiritual or Religious? 18
Unhealthy Guilt as Soul Sickness 19
Healing Soul Sickness 22

CHAPTER TWO/*Guilt, Shame, and Self-Esteem* 26

Healthy Guilt 26
Shame as an Innate Response (Healthy Shame) 28
Shame as a False Identity (Unhealthy Shame) 30
Shame and Spirituality 31
Know Thyself 32
Twenty-one Expressions of Unhealthy Guilt 35
Unhealthy Guilt and Adult Children of Alcoholics 43
Shame and Self-Esteem 45
Overcoming the Tyranny of Black-and-White Thinking 47
Suggestions for the Reader 49

CHAPTER THREE/*The Inner Child's Drama* 50

Conditional and Unconditional Love 51
The Interpersonal Bridge 52

Shame and Broken Bridges: Stephanie's Childhood 54
The Mask: Psychological and Spiritual Models of the False Self . 57
The Shadow: The Long Bag We Drag Behind Us 62
A Summary of the Inner Child's Drama 65
The Inner Child's Guidance 68
Suggestions for the Reader 69

CHAPTER FOUR/*Healing the Inner Child* 70

Letting Bound Emotions Out of the Bag 71
Inner Wisdom Exercises for Healing the Inner Child 72
Exercise: Restoring Bridges to the Inner Child 72
Exercise: Visiting the Inner Child on a Regular Basis 74
Illness and the Inner Child 75
Learning to Listen 78
Love's Epilogue on Growing Up 80
Suggestions for the Reader 82

PART TWO/*Spiritual Beginnings* 83

CHAPTER FIVE/*Who Am I?* 85

The Many Me's 87
The I That Doesn't Change 90
Searching for the Self: The Hero's Journey 91
Psychospiritual Aspects of Myth and Symbol 93
Natural Experiences of the Self: The Enchantment of the Heart . 96
Learning to Experience the Self 98
Basic Meditation 100
The Power of Ritual Centering 105
Dreams and Intuition 106
Suggestions for the Reader 113

CHAPTER SIX/*Spiritual ReVision: A Nation of Closet Mystics* . . 115

Looking Within 116
A Nation of Closet Mystics 119
Religion or Spirituality? 120
Religious Guilt 123

Spiritual ReVision 126
Enlightenment and the Dark Night of the Soul 129
Grace 131
Grace, Love, and Awareness 134
Suggestions for the Reader 137

CHAPTER SEVEN/*From Religious Guilt to Spiritual Optimism* . 138

Why Do Bad Things Happen? 140
Guilt: The Interface Between Psychology and Religion 143
Religious Guilt and Spiritual Pessimism 145
The Shadow of Spiritual Pessimism 147
New Age Philosophy and Spiritual Pessimism 147
New Age Guilt 150
Original Sin or Original Blessing? Traditions of Spiritual Optimism 153
The Prodigal Son—A Parable of Spiritual Optimism 155
The Union of Psychological and Spiritual Wisdom 157
Spiritually Optimistic Transformations 159
Suggestions for the Reader 168

PART THREE/*Compassion: The Flower of Psychospiritual Growth* 169

CHAPTER EIGHT/*Forgiveness* 171

Compassion 172
Forgiveness 174
The Two Sides of Forgiveness 176
The Steps to Forgiving Ourselves 177
The Steps to Forgiving Others 183
Self-Acceptance, Pride, and Humility 187
Forgiveness as an Attitude of Nonjudgmentalness 189
Suggestions for the Reader 190

CHAPTER NINE/*Relationships* 192

Love's Promise—A Preview of Coming Attractions 193
I Am Who I Am. You Are Who You Are 194

Who's to Blame? 195
The Story of David and Sandy 197
The Male and Female Aspects 198
Growing Up Together 200
Giving and Receiving 203
Full Circle to Our Parents 205
Suggestions for the Reader 210

CHAPTER TEN/*Spiritual Exercises and Resources* 211

Practices of Remembering 212
Touchstones for Remembering 213
Inner Wisdom Exercises (Guided Meditations) 215
Reading List 222
On Audiocassette: Joan's Tapes 226
Services Provided by Joan's Organization 227
On Videocassette 228
Psychospiritual Growth Groups 228
Education and Information 229
And in Parting 230

Index 233

A Personal Introduction to Guilt and Healing

This is a book about remembering what we have lost. How many times have you awakened in the morning, groaning about the prospect of a new day with all its chores, anxieties, and difficulties? How many times has your mind reviewed yesterday's regrets and anticipated tomorrow's fears before the new day has even begun? Mornings when we greet the world with weariness and worry are a poignant reminder of what most of us lose as we grow older—the natural state of curiosity, wonder, gratitude, and enthusiasm that makes children so delightful.

I remember how special it was to pick up my children from their cribs in the morning, when they were so full of vitality about the day to come. Living in the present moment, they approached life with wonder, anticipation, and honesty. If they were hungry or wet, they cried or screamed. If they were content, they laughed and smiled. They were authentically human and free to express themselves in a way that adults often cannot. As we grow older, our duties, responsibilities, and roles too often assume control of us. No longer free to express our moods, needs, and fantasies, many of us find our security in the act of pleasing others. Our natural moods and impulses feel shameful, and we gradually learn to block them out, resigned to live in a state of unhealthy guilt where the futile effort to please everyone, do good, be "perfect," and keep ourselves safe and secure in the process keeps us prisoners of the urge to do what we think we "should" do. In saying yes to guilt, we begin saying no to life.

The fullness of what I had lost to guilt became suddenly clear to me one night several years ago. It was early winter, and I was in the midst of an all too frequent "crunch" at work. I had been ministering to endless patients, helping friends in need, and trying to keep up with my research. Getting up at 5:30 or 6:00 A.M. each day to exercise and meditate gave me the illusion that I was taking time for myself even though I was chronically exhausted. I had no illusions about the fact that there wasn't enough time for my family. I felt guilty and stressed. Despite half-hearted efforts to slow down, I was trapped. The merry-go-round was spinning too fast to step off. Even though I tried to hide from my feelings, I was unhappy. The stage was set for disaster.

Driving home late one night in a state of near-total exhaustion, I was suddenly roused by the unforgettable squeal of tires and burning brakes. I was about to have a head-on collision. A short time later, near midnight in the early December darkness, the ambulance with flashing lights and shrieking sirens that always carries away some other unfortunate person brought me back to the hospital where I'd worked for so many years. Two orderlies unloaded me into the emergency room, strapped down to a trauma board in case my spinal cord was injured, which, thank God, it was not. Miraculously, the driver of the other car was able to leave the hospital with minor injuries shortly after being examined. Fortunately, I, too, was nearly unscathed, save for one small part of my anatomy. My nose had been literally destroyed—opened like the hood of a car and nearly torn off my face—when my shoulder harness failed to catch.

"How bad is it?" I asked the surgeon as he finished inspecting the damage. "On a scale of one to ten, ten being the worst," I added, in hopes of regaining some control, at least in the form of concrete information.

"For you," he replied, "it's a one. You're in no danger and will recover completely. For your nose, it's an eight. I haven't seen anything this bad in years."

My heart sank. "Will it work again? Can you put it back together?"

"I think so. I hope so," he replied, adding, "Do you believe in God?" I told him that I did. "Well, He was certainly watching out for you tonight. It's a miracle that only your nose was hurt. Why don't you say a prayer?" He then smiled down at me with great kindness, injected the anesthetic, and began the painstaking process of rearranging a nose from its shattered parts.

A wise man on whom the metaphor of my accident was not lost, the surgeon talked to me seriously about "life in the fast lane." There on the operating table, defenses down, I became acquainted with parts of myself I was still trying to deny, but that were as clear as the nose on my face to the doctor. For years, he had observed me at a distance, rushing through the hospital corridors by day and often leaving for home late at night. Upon reflection, I had to admit that I had sometimes used powerful mind/body techniques to permit me to do too much and run too fast. I had cured the headaches and high blood pressure that once warned me about my stress, removing the fail-safe mechanisms nature had provided.

The period I spent at home recovering from the surgery was a bittersweet time of introspection and redecision. It was a time of seeing the world through new eyes and understanding more deeply what I had lost in leading a life dominated by "unhealthy guilt," a concept we will explore in this book. It was wonderful to be home when my children returned from school and to share little things—missed spelling words, a nice comment from the teacher, or the spat of the day. It was great to have time to cook and read and visit friends. But it was also painful—not physically, but emotionally—as I struggled with the question of why this bad thing had happened. I came to believe that I had a choice. I could see the accident optimistically, as an act of grace inviting me to heal myself on a deeper level. Or I could see it pessimistically, as evidence that, despite all my accomplishments, my deepest fears were true, and I was a failure as a human being.

I chose the optimistic alternative and took advantage of that cosmic punch in the nose to change my life. But first I had to take an honest look at the heavy burden of guilt I had been carrying. Despite years of academic achievement, a curriculum vitae full of research papers, and a thriving clinical practice at a Harvard teaching hospital, nothing I did ever seemed quite "good enough" to me. Despite years of meditation, therapy, and inner discovery, I still felt insecure. I was always apologizing for myself and hoping I wouldn't do anything to make anyone angry. Guilt was my middle name, although I would have denied it to the death—which is what I almost did.

My accident poked a hole in "business as usual," making room for a new point of view. Like most of the cancer and AIDS patients I worked with at the Mind/Body Clinic I had directed for several years, I discovered the value of confronting mortality. With death staring me in the eye, priorities became crystal clear. I was an instant convert to the simple reality that the most important things in life are the three Fs: faith, family, and friends. That's where the love is. Six months after the accident, I finally found the courage to leave my busy job and the academic security it provided. My husband and I founded a business combining our expertise in medical sciences, behavioral medicine, psychology, and spiritual growth.

Our company's bottom line is our own—to promote the healing of society through the healing of individuals. And that healing begins at home. So, although we provide public workshops and seminars, train professionals, and consult to businesses, we do it within limits that leave plenty of room for the three Fs.

My problem with unhealthy guilt and the unhappiness it created for me is far from unique. I recognized guilt's prodding—to do more, do better, save the world, and please everyone—in many of my co-workers. I recognized it for years, in most of my patients, as a common problem we can too easily ignore or rationalize away. That is why it was so hard to take it seriously in myself. "After all," we may think, "isn't everyone else guilty much of the time, too?" Unfortunately, many of us are. And it is killing us, if not in body, then surely in spirit. I received a humorous confirmation of my observations when I began to tell people that I was writing a book about guilt. The most common responses were, "Thank God. Please hurry!" and "Quick, mail a copy to my mother!"

For those of you who have been waiting a long time for this book, I am delighted that I survived my guilt to share some of my ongoing journey of healing with you. I believe passionately that we heal as a world through sharing our struggles, our wounds, our victories, our hopes, and our dreams. Thornton Wilder said, "Without your wounds where would your power be? The very angels themselves cannot persuade the wretched and blundering children on earth as can one human being broken in the wheels of living. In love's service, only the wounded soldiers can serve." It is in this spirit that I offer this book to you.

You may be surprised at the breadth of what we will explore together in the pages to come. The subject of unhealthy guilt is a fascinating one that ultimately involves concerns much deeper than the mind, the body, and our individual pasts. Recovering from guilt is a spiritual search as much as a psychological one. In the following pages, we will share insights from science, philosophy, medicine, psychology, the ancient spiritual texts, the lives of mystics, and the incredibly rich stories of our lives, as we explore together the age-old question that guilt asks of us: Who am I?

The question of who we are spans three spheres of knowledge reflected in the organization of the book. Part One examines the *temporal realm* of space and time circumscribed by our personal, psychological history. Part Two explores the *eternal realm* of soul and spirit in which we live *now*, whether or not we're aware of its influence on our lives. Part Three explores the *realm of relationship* that informs and unites our psychological and spiritual selves through the development of compassion and the practice of forgiveness.

The first sphere of knowledge is psychological. Understanding the psychology of guilt and shame is the starting point for healing. In the childhood need to please parents and keep safe, the developing psyche splits into a public self, or mask, and a private self, or shadow, unknown even to ourselves. In this split, we lose our authentic sense of self and the ability to express our natural impulses. We lose the peace and power that are our birthrights. We become anxious, guilty, empty of vitality, and prone to thinking and acting like victims, and often we become physically ill.

We heal by *remembering*, literally bringing back into the wholeness of our being that which we have lost by hiding it from ourselves. The recovery of awareness and acceptance of *all* emotions as valid messengers about our interaction with the world is the starting point for healing our self-concept. Repairing our relationship to ourself can be aided substantially by discovering and working with the inner children of our past who continue to influence our thoughts, feelings, and actions as adults. Later on in this book, we will do some of this inner child work together.

The second sphere of knowledge is spiritual. We glimpse it through intuition, "holy moments" when the world suddenly stands still and we feel connected to some Greater Spirit, and through love, the interpersonal bridge between two souls. We glimpse it through dreams, the collective memories of soul growth called myths, personal visions, and mystical experiences that are the norm for many Americans rather than the exception, according to national surveys. These glimpses often lead to *spiritual optimism*, an "inner knowing" that the universal energy is love, that our mistakes are occasions for learning rather than damnation, and that life's darkest passages can be opportunities to realize that love. While religions evolved as a way to connect us to the spiritual, they often fail to do so. Worse still, religious beliefs based on judgmental or punitive "God" figures can be psychologically debilitating, inducing what I call *spiritual pessimism*. The New Age notion of "*creating* our own reality" rather than *participating* in that creation is no less pessimistic. It paves the way for guilt by confusing a pathological desire to control our destiny with the responsibility for living our lives authentically, which yields so many rewards.

The third sphere of knowledge concerns relationship. Relationship is both a psychological and spiritual opportunity when it is based on compassion—the shared bond of empathic understanding that replaces the duality of *I* and *thee* with the unity of *we*. That unity leads to ever-deepening wisdom, both psychological and spiritual, when it is lived in the present-centered way of life called forgiveness. Forgiveness is not a lack of discrimination whereby we let all the criminals out of prison; it is an attitude that permits us to relate to the pain that led to their errors and recognize their need for love. Whereas judgmentalism focuses on flaws, forgiveness focuses on wholeness. As we learn to act from the sphere of forgiveness in all our relationships, we become conduits for a greater energy, a lifeforce that we vibrantly "feel" as love, peace, compassion, power, wisdom, and an enthusiastic gratitude for life.

This book of remembering is based on psychology, science, philosophy, and medicine, as well as the more intimate, personal stories of our lives. In all case histories and examples other than those pertaining to me and my family, I have changed names and any identifying characteristics to protect privacy and provide anonymity. At times, the stories of two or three different people have been combined in a composite. I hope that I have done justice to these stories and preserved the dignity and spirit they embody. In reading these stories and allowing them to merge with, call forth, and hopefully illuminate your own story, you may find that new paths to healing have opened for you. Healing is usually a painful process because it entails looking at our dark sides and our worst fears. But it is by grappling with darkness that we eventually find light, and our pain may be transmuted to wisdom and joy.

To commit ourselves to healing our guilt is to seek, find, and celebrate our essential humanity in a world that too often seems to be a place of purposeless suffering. In using that suffering as a catalyst for renewed self-awareness, we may ultimately discover our true nature as an expression of a Greater Spirit. When our experience convinces us that an eternal harvest of peace, wisdom, love, and joy arises from the temporal seeds of our problems, we can take courage. This hope and promise was stated well by the poet John Keats:

Some say that the world is a vale of tears.
I say it is a place of soul making.

Healing our guilt is an opportunity for soul making.

—Scituate, Massachusetts
June 21, 1989
Summer Solstice

PART ONE

Psychological Beginnings

You are not alone in your struggles
nor will you ever be alone.
From the beginning of time the human heart
has sought its source in love.
Guilt is one of many guides back to that source.

We can love and help one another
only as we have been loved ourselves.
So the fear, the "sins" of the father
are visited on the child
who forgets his birthright of uniqueness and joy
falling asleep to the love that he is.

The journey of awakening
is a remembering of Who we really are
where fear is cured by love
and the mask we have worn to purchase affection
melts away in the willingness to rejoice
in our shadow as well as our light.

Only then can we pick up our power and move on
to a connectedness with caring, compassion and love
where we can sing our own songs with joy and thanksgiving
exulting in our worthiness
as children of God.

—J. B.

CHAPTER ONE

Bodymind and Soul: A Psychospiritual Perspective on Guilt

I used to think that making a mistake was the worst thing on earth. Mistakes meant I wasn't good enough and people wouldn't like me. I might be ridiculed, rejected, or abandoned. Making a mistake meant that I would immediately forget all the good things I'd ever done and focus on that one error until it seemed to become the totality of who I was.

Mistakes were an open invitation to self-criticism, anxiety, depression, paranoia, and even panic. The omnipresent fear of error created physical tension, stress, frequent illness, and a pervasive sense in me that the other shoe was about to drop. It created a kind of *unhealthy guilt* that bore no relation to the genuine and important remorse of *healthy guilt* that teaches us conscience by providing emotional feedback about the consequences of hurtful behavior.

Unhealthy guilt made me feel bad about almost everything I did because, after all, I could have done a better job. Having to be perfect made it hard for me to take risks and stifled my creativity. It made me competitive, tight-lipped, defensive, and awfully serious about myself. It made for constant comparisons between me and others, during which I always worried about being one up or one down. It made me hypersensitive to criticism, which I heard even where it wasn't intended. I was like a fortress constantly prepared for attack.

Worse still, I was angry much of the time (and nice people shouldn't be angry, right?). Unable to forgive myself or anyone else, I was a prisoner of guilt and resentment. I did my best to hide all this underneath a smile but was ultimately betrayed by my body, which became a breeding ground for stress-related illnesses ranging from high blood pressure and migraine headaches to a spastic colon and constant respiratory infections. Throughout the book, I will present many stories of patients whose guilt culminated in physical, emotional, and spiritual distress, but a fuller look at the genesis of my own problem seems like a good place to start.

THE BODYMIND

Born in Boston at the end of the Second World War, I was a goody-goody for most of my childhood. I remember being stood up on an umbrella table under the bright summer sun to sing a song for relatives when I was very small. Even though painfully shy, I psyched myself up to perform before all those expectant faces that seemed to loom as large as bugs do under a microscope. It would never, never have occurred to me to say no. I did what I was asked. Throughout grammar school, I tutored the other children in reading, knit intricate cablework sweaters, and was the first one on my block to get a Red Cross Swimmer's card. My brother claims I had my homework done a month in advance! (He exaggerates, but only slightly.)

I was, however, a lousy ballet dancer. You have to be able to relax and let go to dance well, but I was too frightened of making a mistake. I still can remember how a classmate, that red-haired Charlotte with the big feet and the graceful pirouettes, laughed herself silly when my best effort landed me in a twisted heap on the studio floor. My pride was injured worse than my derriere. My face turned the color of her hair, and I felt unmasked, revealed as a hopelessly inferior and worthless creature. I wished that the floor would open up and swallow me. I experienced the emotion we call shame, which accompanies the sudden vulnerability and threatening feelings we experience whenever the bridge of trust and acceptance between us and others is suddenly broken.

I begged my mother to let me quit ballet lessons, but they were part of the plan for proper little ladies of the fifties. Week after week, I went to class feeling like a dismal failure. It seemed as though one hundred eyes were on me when I performed my tense, stiff pliés. Even now I can feel my breath get shallow and stop as I remember how small and isolated I felt. I didn't like or trust myself, and most of my energy went into trying to impress the other children. Ironically, the harder I tried to control the situation, the more I fell on my face—literally. I usually had a pounding, nerve-shattering headache by the time I got home.

Sometimes I actually appreciated the frequent migraine headaches I suffered. At least they kept me out of ballet class from time to time! In early childhood I had discovered "stress" and its contribution to illness. By the time I was twenty-four years old and a graduate student in medical sciences at Harvard Medical School, the combined stress of academic pressure, a marriage that was on the rocks, and the sudden pressures of caring for an infant son overwhelmed me. My body responded with more migraines, high blood pressure, panic attacks, irritable bowel syndrome, chronic bronchitis, fainting spells, and assorted aches and pains. A fellow student reasoned that my symptoms would disappear when I learned to relax and encouraged me to practice yoga and meditation. These mind/body skills saved my life physically at first, and then led more slowly to the psychological and spiritual recovery that are still underway for me.

Understanding the mind/body connection psychologically, physically, and spiritually became the focus of my life's work, both personally and professionally. In my first book, *Minding the Body, Mending the Mind*, I shared part of my own ongoing journey of healing and some of the journeys of the thousands of people who sought help for stress-related disorders and chronic illness at the Mind/Body Clinic. I cofounded the clinic and then directed it for six years at two different Harvard teaching hospitals, in the hospitals' Behavioral Medicine sections, under the aegis of Dr. Herbert Benson. Our clinic was originally modeled on a program pioneered by Dr. Jon Kabat-Zinn, the Stress Reduction and Relaxation Program at the University of Massachusetts Medical School.

In the Mind/Body Clinic, which still operates in the Section on Behavioral Medicine at Boston's New England Deaconess Hospital, some patients come with illnesses either caused by or worsened by stress, such as ulcers, irritable bowel syndrome, migraine headaches, insomnia, asthma, high blood pressure, pain, and fatigue. Other people have acute or chronic illnesses like cancer or multiple sclerosis that create stress. In ten weekly two-hour sessions, people are taught to use their minds to change their bodies. After all, a single thought like, "I'll never finish this book and then I'll really be in trouble" can get the nervous system into quite an uproar. Just typing those words tensed my shoulders, raised my heart rate, catapulted my breathing into a fast, shallow, and irregular rhythm, and sent my blood pressure soaring!

Fearful thoughts create the fight-or-flight response that evolved to protect us from danger by providing energy for defense or escape. The fight-or-flight response is like the overdrive on a car. It comes in handy to get us out of occasional tight spots, but if we keep the car in overdrive all the time, the wear and tear on its parts will cause a variety of mechanical problems. In people, these problems are commonly called stress or anxiety-related disorders.

Once, during a course in biofeedback I took several years ago, I experienced a powerful demonstration of how fearful, insecure thinking affects the body. The instructor had a machine similar to a lie-detector test that registered your degree of tension or relaxation by monitoring electrical activity on the skin's surface. The more the activity, the more fight-or-flight was registering, and you could see your state instantly revealed on a dial. When the instructor hooked up a man named John as a demonstration and asked "What's your name?" his response caused no change to register on the dial. Similarly, answers to the questions "Where do you live" and "What kind of work do you do?" provoked no response on the machine.

In order to get a rise out of John, the instructor finally asked, "What are your sexual fantasies like?" As we all giggled nervously, John's fight-or-flight circuit finally engaged and up went the needle on the dial! It was my turn next. I felt all eyes watching. "What's your name?" the instructor asked. And that's all it took. The dial practically fell off the machine! I was treated, in public, to the realization that my fight-or-flight system went on the defensive to any inquiry at all. My whole purpose in life apparently revolved around defending myself. Although I would have been the last person to admit it (because, like many guilty people, I could not see it), I was ruled by fear. Fear is the very heart of unhealthy guilt. Learning to turn off the fight-or-flight system is the first step in recovery from guilt.

In the 1940s, the Nobel prize–winning physiologist Walter Hesse discovered that he could produce two diametrically opposed energy states by stimulating different areas in the hypothalamus of the cat. One state was the high-energy fight-or-flight response; the other was a state of low energy expenditure characterized by deep rest and relaxation. More recently, Drs. R. Keith Wallace and Herbert Benson documented a similar state of profound rest in humans who practiced transcendental meditation. Benson went on to show that this state of profound rest accompanied any form of mental concentration that distracted individuals from their usual worries, fears, and concerns. He called this innate hypothalamic mechanism the relaxation response.

When the relaxation response is evoked, stress is reduced. Heart rate and blood pressure drop. Respiratory rate and oxygen consumption decline because of the decrease in the body's need for energy. Brain waves shift from an alert beta rhythm to a relaxed alpha and theta rhythm. Blood flow to the muscles decreases; instead, blood is sent to the brain and skin, producing a feeling of warmth and rested alertness where mental cobwebs seem to melt away. The tissues of the body actually become less sensitive to the stress hormone adrenaline, and the immune system is activated. The body is at peace. The mind is also at peace. Thoughts slow down, and there is a feeling of contentment and comfort.

Participants in the Mind/Body Clinic learn to shift into the relaxation response mode by using the breathing techniques, meditation, and guided imagery I described in detail in *Minding the Body, Mending the Mind*. The benefits of these techniques are quite remarkable, not only for the body but also for the mind, and especially for the soul and its connection to the Spirit, which we will explore together in the chapters that follow. In the clinic, we begin learning these techniques before looking at the thinking patterns that disrupted the body's natural balance to start with.

The more I listened and learned from patients at the clinic and the thousands of people who have attended my workshops across the country, the more convinced I became that a majority of people with stress-related disorders are actually suffering from the same emotion that afflicted me in ballet class—an inner feeling of unworthiness that generates an impressive array of coping strategies all aimed at self-protection. As we'll see, the seemingly unitary person we think of as "me" is actually more like a committee of subpersonalities, each doing its best to keep us safe from situations that threatened us in the past. While our bodies and intellects grow to adulthood, most of us still harbor the emotional ghosts of ourselves as children, frightened and insecure like little Joanie tripping over her feet in ballet. Healing our guilt involves putting these ghosts to rest by giving them the love they need to let go of their self-protective fear.

Mind/body techniques can be used as a key to healing guilt. They are useful on several levels that build on and reinforce each other. At a basic body level, they elicit the relaxation response and act like a medication to turn down the fight-or-flight system and restore balance to the body. At a psychological level, they act as a powerful system to promote self-awareness. Even the simple practice of closing your eyes, taking a few deep breaths and mentally scanning your body for areas of tension, relaxation, high energy, and low energy expands your awareness of your inner state and allows you to make a conscious choice to relax or re-energize areas of tension. Similarly, as I discussed in *Minding the Body, Mending the Mind*, meditation leads to awareness of emotions that may not usually be noticed, as well as habitual patterns of thinking that create suffering.

In the chapters that follow, we will use meditation and imagery exercises to produce the relaxation response and to increase self-awareness and self-acceptance. We will also use these techniques to contact the committee of frightened inner children whose fear has long ceased to serve us. In understanding and comforting these often-forgotten parts of ourself, we can heal shame and the unhealthy guilt, stress, and illness it creates. This inner work encompasses but goes beyond the physiological effects of meditation, producing a deeper level of healing by touching our psychological core.

While the physical and psychological levels of mind/body healing are extremely powerful, they attain their full benefit only when combined with an entity that is generally left out of both medical and psychological treatment. That entity is *soul*, our personal reflection of the Spirit or Lifeforce that is the energy from which mind and body arise. Without considering soul and Spirit, our healing from guilt and the stress, anxiety, helplessness, depression, and physical symptoms it creates cannot be complete. As one of my patients expressed it, "I've had eight years of therapy and the best medical treatment, but there's a place inside me that nothing has touched." That place is the soul, and our healing must go deep enough to reach it. While the relation between body, mind, Spirit, and guilt will be explored in depth in Part Two, I want to introduce some key concepts about soul, Spirit, and healing before we take a closer look at the psychology of guilt.

SOUL AND SPIRIT—INDIVIDUAL CONSCIOUSNESS OR ONE MIND?

The word *psychology* derives from the Greek *psyche* and *logos* and means "study of the soul," but psychology has traditionally concerned itself with study of the mind. The original separation of medicine and then psychology from the study of the soul stemmed from the necessity of healers to avoid conflicts with beliefs held by the early Christian church. For example, Christian Orthodoxy strictly forbade dissection of the human body and so the great medical schools of the Middle Ages were located in Persia where Islam and Judaism tolerated it. At a time when death for heresy and witchcraft was a common punishment in Christian Europe, scientists and physicians quickly learned to leave the soul to theologians, lest they be denounced as witches or devils in their practice of the healing arts. Physicians became technicians of the body, psychologists technicians of the mind, and clergy the sometimes jealous keepers of the soul.

This artificial separation of mind, body, and spirit reached its fullest expression in the twentieth century. Dr. Larry Dossey, a physician, lecturer, and writer, refers to the practice of medicine over the past hundred years as Era I, or "materialistic medicine," in which:

> . . . the emphasis is on the material body, which is viewed largely as a complex machine. Era I medicine is guided by the laws of energy and matter laid down by Newton three hundred years ago. According to this perspective the universe and all in it—including the body—are a vast clockwork functioning according to deterministic principles. The effects of mind and consciousness are absent, and all forms of therapy must be physical in nature—drugs, surgery, irradiation, etc.
>
> —*Recovering the Soul*

Era I medicine has unquestionably improved the quality and length of life. After all, vitamins are a relatively recent discovery, as were antibiotics, which came into use only at the time of the Second World War. Without them, many of us would not be alive today. Technological advances in surgery and pharmacology have been truly incredible. As I sometimes joke, I would hate to have had to meditate my nose back onto my face after the accident! I am deeply grateful to my surgeon's skill and to the technology that supported it.

About twenty years ago, however, the limitations of Era I medicine began to become apparent. As miraculous as its achievements were, they often proved insufficient. Patient statistics showed that up to 90 percent of the reason for visits to the family doctor were for "stress" or anxiety-related problems. While pills might provide temporary relief, they were merely Band-Aids, since the real cause of the illness wasn't addressed. This was exactly the problem I experienced two decades ago when I sought help for my headaches, stomach pain, high blood pressure, and chronic bronchitis. Pills provided only limited relief. It wasn't until I began to use a mind/body approach that relied on powerful meditation and imagery techniques, combined with insight into the attitudes that put my body out of balance to begin with, that I began to heal.

The scientific research of the last twenty years is replete with examples of mind/body interactions. If our hospital room looks out on a tree, we heal faster than if it faces a brick wall. If we are lonely, our immune systems and our hearts suffer. Men who smoke are more likely to die sooner if divorced, widowed, or single than if they are married. This research suggests that the mind and body are not separate entities, but a single unit, the bodymind, which responds physically as well as emotionally to the presence of other bodyminds and to nature itself.

Dossey calls the advent of mind/body medicine, used in conjunction with appropriate mechanistic approaches, Era II medicine. But even Era II medicine has inherent limitations because it is based on the concept of an isolated bodymind unit—a single consciousness residing in a single body—which may be influenced by, but is inherently unconnected to, any other source of consciousness. Consciousness, or mind, is assumed to be a function of the brain. When the brain dies, so does consciousness.

I had occasion to doubt this assumption many years ago when I sat with a young woman who was dying. Her name was Sally, and she had been living with a rapidly growing and rare rectal cancer for the year or so that we knew each other. We worked on meditation and imagery techniques that helped relieve treatment side effects and brought Sally some peace. We talked of emotions, finishing old business, forgiveness, and grieving. We also talked about Sally's concept of death, which was the Era I perspective—that consciousness died with the brain rather than surviving in any way beyond the body.

When the day of Sally's death came, I was visiting her in the hospital. I was scared because I'd never been with a dying person before and didn't have any notion of what to expect. Her parents had gone off to have lunch when I came, so I had about forty-five minutes to sit alone with Sally. To my great relief, she seemed comfortable as she drifted in and out of consciousness. We just sat together in the silence. Then after a while I screwed up my courage and asked, "Where do you drift off to, Sally? Your face looks so peaceful." She opened her eyes and turned to look at me. Her eyes were full of love and wonder.

In a tiny, soft, and very amused voice, she said, "Well, you may have trouble believing this, but I've been floating around, touring the hospital. I've just been to the cafeteria, watching my parents eat lunch. Dad is having grilled cheese. Mom is eating tuna. They are so sad they can barely eat. I will have to tell them that my body may be dying, but *I'm* certainly not. It's more like I'm being born—my consciousness is so free and peaceful." Sally faded out for a while and when she came back she told me, "It's so *beautiful*, Joan. I'm drifting up out of my body toward a kind of living light. It's very bright. So *warm*, so loving." She squeezed my hand a little, "Don't be afraid to die," she said looking at me with so much kindness. "Your soul doesn't die at all. You know? It just goes home. It just goes on from here."

That moment of looking into Sally's eyes as she shared the beginning of her soul's journey out of her physical body held a special magic for me. It is one of the highlights of my life. Sally's experience—that her individual consciousness, or soul, was not bound to her body—lies at the core of most spiritual traditions. The purpose of spiritual life is to recollect that our seemingly separate soul is not separate at all, but part of a Greater Spirit—in the poet Kahlil Gibran's words, one of the "sons and daughters of life's longing for itself." In that realization, that *remembrance* of its oneness with the Source of Life, the soul is mended —healed from its temporal sorrows as it remembers its true identity as wisdom, consciousness, and love.

The personal experiences of people like Sally, which we will discuss in greater depth in Part Two, have begun a revolution in thinking that has challenged the most dearly held tenets of medicine, psychology, and religion. Data from well-controlled scientific studies further challenged our assumptions about the nature of mind and how we can affect one another through shared consciousness. Cardiologist Randolph Byrd, for example, demonstrated that patients admitted to the coronary intensive care unit with heart attacks fared significantly better medically if they were prayed for than if they were not! Since patients in Byrd's studies were randomly assigned to either the prayed-for or non-prayed-for group, and neither staff nor patients knew which group they were in, the results could not be accounted for by suggestion. In a similar vein, data from more than thirty studies conducted by scientists studying transcendental meditation revealed a significant decrease in crime and violence in cities where 1 percent or more of the population were meditators.

How is it that our minds can affect one another at a distance? The mechanistic concept of one mind in one body that has informed medicine and psychology for the last century cannot explain such phenomena. Dossey suggests that the medicine of the future, Era III medicine, will include the spiritual dimension that recognizes the Greater Mind of which we are all a part.

Prayer and meditation are most fully utilized not only as techniques to promote physical healing, but also as a means of rediscovering our connection with that Greater Mind. This deeper healing encompasses the perennial questions: What is the meaning of life? Who am I? What is consciousness? What is Divinity? What is a human life well lived? Medicine, psychology, and spirituality intersect in the answers to these questions, which have traditionally been the purview of religion. Religion, as we'll consider in Chapter Seven, has been deeply influenced by, and in some cases corrupted by, worldviews based on guilt.

SPIRITUAL OR RELIGIOUS?

Here I would like to make an important distinction between Religion and Spirituality. For me, the difference is best expressed in the following comment by a good friend of mine, physician and psychotherapist Rachel Naomi Remen. She says:

> The spiritual is not the religious. A religion is a dogma, a set of beliefs about the spiritual and a set of practices which rise out of those beliefs. There are many religions and they tend to be mutually exclusive. That is, every religion tends to think that it has dibs on the spiritual—that it's "The Way." Yet the spiritual is inclusive. It is the deepest sense of belonging and participation. . . . One might say that the spiritual is that realm of human experience which religion attempts to connect us to through dogma and practice. Sometimes it succeeds and sometimes it fails. *Religion is a bridge to the spiritual, but the spiritual lies beyond religion* [italics added].

Religions that most easily reconnect us to the divine are based on a psychology and philosophy of *spiritual optimism* that we will consider closely later in the book. Religions that try to control us by generating fear—that we are evil, that we may lose our souls, and that only they (or the particular manifestation of Spirit that they worship) can save us—create *spiritual pessimism* that feeds fear, soul sickness, unworthiness, and guilt. These beliefs are dangerous to our psychological and physical health. Although medicine and psychology have steered clear of religion for most of the last two thousand years, I believe it is time we reunite them in order to promote a new psychology of spiritual optimism that will be a true healer of body, mind, and soul.

An excellent example of how spirituality can intersect with medicine on the common ground of guilt presented itself to me at the Mind/Body Clinic. During my tenure there, I worked with a thirty-seven-year-old patient named Bob who continued to suffer from severe migraines, even though he had made extensive changes in his life. Meditating at least three times a week and running several miles a day, he had given up alcohol, sugar, caffeine, and the occasional marijuana he smoked. I admired his discipline and responsibility, but still the headaches remained a problem. Something was missing.

I finally asked Bob, "What do you think the meaning of life is?" Fascinated and thoughtful, Bob promptly turned to religion. He had been raised by strict and rigidly Catholic parents who were terrified of sin and talked about God as a fearsome judge. The confessional was particularly traumatic to Bob because he felt threatened rather than relieved as he reviewed his "sinful" deeds before a priest. He had questioned and finally rejected his childhood religious upbringing years before I met him. Nonetheless, he told me that he still believed deeply in "some kind of Higher Power," although he didn't think about it much. As he described this Higher Power, it emerged as a kind of malevolent Santa Claus who rewarded good behavior and punished bad. Bob had left his childhood religion behind, but clearly it had never left him.

Bob characterized himself as a "recovering Catholic." Although many people raised in Catholicism have had positive, loving experiences, Bob did not. The combination of his parents' attitude, the strictness of the nuns who ran his parochial school, and the church's emphasis on hell and damnation during his childhood were devastating to Bob's self-esteem. We might even call Bob a victim of spiritual abuse. Like any type of abuse, Bob's strict and limiting religious upbringing produced the same helpless, pessimistic attitude that characterizes unhealthy guilt. In our sessions together, Bob described for me his ability to ruin just about anything—his marriage, his sales record at work (which was usually excellent but, like all things, could not be "perfect" all of the time), even his children, who "weren't doing well enough in school." Everything was all his fault and hopeless. That was the story of his life. While his unfulfilling life may not have been the direct result of Divine punishment, Bob figured it was at least the result of Divine neglect. Grace had abandoned him while making its rounds.

Bob's psychological pessimism, then, was compounded by his spiritual pessimism. Realizing this, I came to believe that Bob's physical healing would not be complete until he was reconnected to his own inner core of peace and worthiness. His soul was effectively separated from its Source. So I sent Bob to a priest who embodied the philosophy of spiritual optimism. The premise of this philosophy is that human beings are by nature good, a part of Divine consciousness, not bad and in need of redemption. When Bob began to think of himself as good, worthy of his own love, and in eternal connection to a larger Source of love, peace, and wisdom, his headaches finally stopped.

UNHEALTHY GUILT AS SOUL SICKNESS

There is a passage from the spiritually optimistic Christian text and workbook known as the *Course in Miracles* that poses the question, "Do

I want to be right, or do I want to be happy?" One of my patients once remarked, "I want to be right because that's what *makes* me happy."

Right makes us feel safe. It protects us from our fear that we are unworthy of love. This fear and doubt create guilt-driven behaviors as diverse as perfectionism; overachievement; lack of assertiveness; "helper's disease," wherein we care for everyone but ourselves; and addiction to substances like drugs or alcohol or processes like work, religious fanaticism, or falling in "love" that dull the pain of our critical self-doubt. Anxiety and depression—conditions in which we think everything is our fault and believe that life is hopeless—are also symptoms of unhealthy guilt. So is the anger that stems from the aching hurt we feel when we think we are unlovable.

Unhealthy guilt is an autoimmune disease of the soul that causes us to literally reject our own worth as human beings. It is an affliction that robs life of joy. Instead of acting out of love and enthusiasm, we are led to act out of self-protection. *Unhealthy guilt causes life to become organized around the need to avoid fear rather than the desire to share love.* Guilt creates a psychic optical illusion that causes faults and fears to stand out while pleasure and happiness recede into the background. The result is a loss of joy and gratitude that creates fatigue, negativity, and depression. In guilt, we say no to life.

This syndrome of unhealthy guilt, which I will characterize more specifically in the next chapter, has been called by many names. I have mentioned perfectionism and overachievement, but there is also narcissism, the shame or stress-prone personality, the codependent personality, and *mishegus* (plain old craziness, according to my Jewish mother). In psychology, it is known as a *character disorder*, a problem more pervasive than a neurosis because it is woven into the warp and woof of how we think and perceive. Guilt becomes the fabric of who we are rather than a passing aberration such as a neurotic fear of dogs or a phobia about crossing bridges. Character disorders are generally thought of as chronic conditions. We can learn to live with them, but they are usually incurable. Like an addict, we are always in recovery.

I disagree with the finality of this point of view. I believe that unhealthy guilt is curable but that it requires the psychological equivalent of an Era III approach. An Era I intervention such as an antidepressant or other medication may relieve the depression that sometimes accompanies guilt. An Era II approach—some form of self-evaluation and new awareness of the bodymind system, such as reading, journal keeping, or individual group therapy—may also aid the recovery. But these approaches alone are often not enough. As in Bob's case, the spiritual dimension also needs to be included in our healing if we are to cure the equivalent of a chronic illness.

A bell went off in my mind when, in my research, I read a letter that the noted psychiatrist Dr. Carl Jung had written many years ago to Bill W., one of the founders of Alcoholics Anonymous. In it, Jung stated that alcoholism was too deeply seated to be cured by psychological means alone, and that Bill W.'s hopes lay in a "spiritual conversion." Bill W. had that conversion, of course, and out of it was born the twelve-step programs that have been called the greatest spiritual force in America today.

Just as many people have been grateful for their alcoholism, because recovering from it has led them to explore life more deeply and find more joy, I have been grateful for my unhealthy guilt. An ancient principle reminds us to look for salvation in the darkest, most painful parts of our lives. We emerge into the light not by denying our pain, but by walking out through it. The common turn of phrase we apply to this wonderful action of grace is: "That was a blessing in disguise." The head-on collision I described in the introduction was such an act of grace. It led me to probe the darkest recesses of myself.

William James, the physician and scientist who fathered American psychology at the turn of the century, coined the term *soul sickness* to describe the syndrome of unhealthy guilt, chronic stress, perfectionism, and its associated physical symptoms. Like Jung, he emphasized the need for man's spiritual conversion, a total reconsideration of our place in the Universe, in order for there to be a cure from soul sickness and a return to a state he called *healthy mindedness*.

In 1901, James was invited to give the prestigious Gifford lectures on religion at the University of Edinburgh, the cardinal honor bestowed on philosophers in his time. The lecture series was published as the enduring classic *The Varieties of Religious Experience*. In that work, James discusses the "New Thought" movement begun by Dr. Phineas Parkhurst Quimby, whose most famous patient, Mary Baker Eddy, went on to advance some of his principles as Christian Science. The New Thought movement of the mid-1800s bears striking similarities to what we now call the New Age movement. Now, as then, there is nothing new about these ideas. They are based on the ancient wisdom that life's purpose lies in realizing the enduring connection of the individual consciousness to the greater Whole—of the soul to the Spirit. James cites a letter written to him by a woman healed by New Thought principles. It sounds remarkably contemporary. The attitude that cured this woman of the physical and psychological symptoms of her soul sickness is a fine description of the spiritual, as opposed to religious, conversion that Carl Jung prescribed as necessary for healing deep-seated addictions or character disorders. The woman writes to James:

> Life seemed difficult to me at one time. I was always breaking down, and had several attacks of what is called nervous prostration, with terrible insomnia, being on the verge of insanity; besides having many other troubles, especially of the digestive organs. I had been sent away from home in charge of doctors, had taken all the narcotics, stopped all work, been fed up, and in fact knew all the doctors within reach. But I never recovered permanently till this New Thought took possession of me.
>
> I think that the one thing which impressed me most was learning the fact that we must be in absolutely constant relation or mental touch (this word is to me very expressive) with that essence of life which permeates all and which we call God. This is almost unrecognizable unless we live it into ourselves *actually*, that is, by a constant turning to the very innermost, deepest consciousness of our real selves or of God in us, for illumination from within, just as we turn to the sun for light, warmth, and invigoration without.

This woman's description of her renewed relationship with the Divine is a wonderful example of a spiritual conversion that was accompanied by physical healing. As we'll see in Chapter Seven, however, *although physical healing is related in some cases to spiritual healing, they are not in any way a direct reflection of one another*. Illumined spiritual teachers die of heart disease and cancer just like the rest of us, while cantankerous pessimists who smoke cigarettes and eat lots of hamburgers sometimes live to be a hundred. And all of us, no matter how many bean sprouts we eat, miles we run, affirmations we say, hours we meditate, and hard we pray, are all going to die sometime. The question is not whether we will die but how we will live.

HEALING SOUL SICKNESS

The following story was passed along to me by a wise friend and former colleague, Steve Maurer, who is current director of the Mind/Body Clinic. It is a joke—or more properly a teaching tale—about two great beings,

Jesus and Moses, on the golf course. I offer this story, with the greatest respect for the Judeo-Christian tradition, as a metaphor for our own healing. As the story begins, Jesus and Moses have teed up at a very long hole, and Jesus is sizing up his golf bag. Unexpectedly, he pulls out a seven iron.

"Jesus, it's a long hole," says Moses. "You'll never make it with a seven iron. Better use a driver."

Jesus smiles and replies, "Arnold Palmer does it." Then he hits the ball with a resounding thwack, and it lands right in the middle of a big water hazard. Moses generously offers to shag the ball and give his friend another crack at it. So Moses saunters over to the water hazard and, with great aplomb, parts the waters and picks out the ball. Jesus tees up again, and again he takes the seven iron.

Moses laments, "Jesus, you already tried that iron. Believe me, the hole is too long. Here's a driver."

Jesus patiently shakes his head and steps up to the ball. "Arnold Palmer does it," he says. Then he hits the ball smartly, and it sails high and short, landing once again in the same hazard. This time Jesus goes off to shag the ball himself. He approaches the hazard, walks across the water, and picks out the ball. Meanwhile, the next foursome of players has caught up from behind and is looking on, astonished,

"Who does he think he is," says one man, "Jesus Christ?"

"No," says Moses sadly. "Unfortunately, he thinks he's Arnold Palmer."

Like the Jesus of this story, many of us lose touch with our own indwelling Divine nature—the unlimited creative potential of love the real Jesus assured us could literally move mountains. Identifying instead with our faults and our desires to be "good," "perfect," or at least acceptable, we look for worth in our achievements. We don different ego masks and postures that make us feel lovable and valued, yet there is still an inner emptiness. Our self-critic is a harsh judge telling us that we are never good enough, never worthy of our own love. In spite of all our achievements, peace and self-acceptance remain elusive, and we are guilty and stressed. *We have forgotten who we really are.*

In the remaining chapters of Part One, we will explore the roots of this case of mistaken identity and see how we can begin to correct it. I believe in my heart that guilt's pain is nothing more than the feedback of grace, an indication that we are searching for our worthiness in the wrong place. We are like the man who was looking for his keys under the streetlamp. When a helpful passerby joined in the search, asking where exactly the keys were lost, the man pointed to a vacant lot across the street. When the passerby asked the obvious question, "Why search for the keys here, then?," the man replied, "Because the light is better."

The recovery from guilt necessarily redirects our search from the outer world to the inner one. We access our real identity, what many philosophies and psychologies call the Self, whenever the mind becomes quiet and we are fully present in the moment. The delight of skiing, sailing, gardening, reading, or being in nature are inherent in us, not in the activity. If we're fearful or preoccupied, even the most delightful pastime loses its savor. But whenever our guard is down—yielding to the majesty of a sunset, the caress of a breeze, the silence of a heartfelt hug—we reexperience the inner current of joy and love that is always present. This Self is like a pebble resting gently on the bottom of a pond. When the waters are turbulent, we cannot see it, but it is there nonetheless.

The search for the Self is identified as the purpose of life in the world's oldest stories. It is told and retold in the myths, fairy tales, and religious metaphors of every culture. In religion, we search for the Kingdom of God, for heaven, and for eternal peace. In myth, we yearn for Camelot, search for the Golden Fleece, and quest for the Holy Grail. As a society, we thrill to the archetype of good and evil sparring to define the world. We gasp as the young Luke Skywalker confronts arch-villain Darth Vader, only to find that he is battling his own father, just as we must battle the dark and hidden aspects of our own natures. We understand in metaphor that our best is cultivated only by confronting darkness.

After all, what else can mobilize us so well, and help us overcome the hypnotic inertia of day-to-day life? Isn't crisis and pain the universal great awakener? In facing our "dark" parts, the disowned parts of our being that we thought were unworthy of love, we learn to live whole, authentic lives. We reown the energy deposited in what Carl Jung called the shadow—the long bag containing discarded parts of our self that we unconsciously drag behind us throughout life. In the shadow, we find the power that allows us to live life with enthusiasm, excitement, and joy—the natural impulses lost from childhood.

In rediscovering the missing parts of ourselves and becoming psychologically whole, we simultaneously mend our souls and become spiritually whole. The flower of psychospiritual growth is loving-kindness and compassion, the ability to suffer *with*, to leave the limited sphere of personal concern and enter into the life of another. In compassion, as we will explore in Chapter Nine, the connection between two souls opens the floodgates through which the Spirit reveals its nature as love and we remember who we really are.

To remember means to rejoin—to reunite. In this life, we are called to reunite the forces of light and darkness, good and evil, public mask and hidden shadow. This is not an easy task. It is what Joseph Campbell called the hero's journey. We are all the potential heros of our own lives. At journey's end, hopefully in this life, we will realize the inner Kingdom. We will remember love as the Source and ground of our being. We will remember our Self as intimately and eternally connected to that Source. The joy, enthusiasm, and creativity that are in us will then be able to express themselves as a gratitude for life, an engagement with life, a yes to life, in its inevitable sorrows as well as its joys.

My hope is that this book will be a remembering for you and that, as we share our stories, you will come to know that you are not alone and, as is said so well in *Emmanuel's Book: A Guide for Living Comfortably in the Cosmos*, compiled by Pat Rodegast and Judith Stanton,

> *There is nothing but love.*
> *Don't let the masks and postures fool you.*
> *Love is the glue*
> *that holds the Universe together.*
> *The greatest need in a soul*
> *is to achieve that loving of self*
> *which will bring about the unity*
> *wherein the judgments*
> *that have caused such pain*
> *are eliminated.*
>
> *True self-love is not ego.*
> *True love is great humility.*
> *Love and compassion for others*
> *cannot exist*
> *until there is a goodly supply for self.*
> *How can you feel the love of God*
> *if you do not love yourself?*
> *Are they not one and the same thing?*

Come, and let us remember together.

CHAPTER TWO

Guilt, Shame, and Self-Esteem

Six patients, two friends, and my husband, Myrin, gave me a clipping from the *Boston Globe* one Sunday that tackled the serious matter of unhealthy guilt in a refreshingly light way. The article was titled "The Guilt Tripper."

The article concerned a man who went to the luggage store to buy a new suitcase for his guilt. The old one was full. The man found just the ticket, a marvelous item designed by a panel of psychiatrists and leather craftsmen. It had compartments for every kind of guilt imaginable, including guilt for working too hard and guilt for goofing off. Guilt for not making enough money and guilt for making too much. Guilt for successful ventures and guilt for failure. I got very excited. I wondered if it had room for some of my favorites like guilt for eating too much chocolate and not enough bean sprouts. Happily, I read on and learned that it had plenty of room for miscellaneous guilt. It even had wheels for dragging it through the airport!

HEALTHY GUILT

Unfortunately, the writer forgot to tell us where he had bought this fabulous invention, but he did set me to thinking that some kinds of guilt are not stored in our burden bags. Some guilt is an asset. It serves our interests.

Consider the story of Jennifer, a student I knew many years ago when I was teaching microscopic anatomy to medical and dental students.

During the first lab quiz of the year, I caught Jennifer trying to eyeball an answer from the student at the next desk. I approached Jennifer and asked her to keep her eyes on her own paper. A few hours later, she appeared at my office, nervous and downcast. In a tremulous voice, Jennifer told me how ashamed she felt for cheating. *This is healthy guilt.*

Insecure about her first test in medical school, Jennifer had let fear overwhelm her judgment. We talked about the pressures of med school, the need to achieve, how to study, and when to ask for help. We also talked about Jennifer's motivation for cheating, which helped her acknowledge and begin to explore the insecurity in which the incident was rooted. Jennifer's healthy guilt and its accompanying psychic pain led her to take responsibility for the incident by admitting that she had cheated, reflecting honestly about why she had done it, understanding what she could do to prevent its recurrence, and resolving that it would not happen again.

This process of responsibility, self-inquiry, and letting go of the past renews and deepens self-respect. It is called forgiveness. Forgiveness creates a shift in perception that permits us to see our mistake as an opportunity to learn rather than as proof of how "bad" we are. As we'll discuss in Part Three, *forgiveness ensures that the fruits of healthy guilt are stored not in our burden bags but in what family therapist Virginia Satir called our wisdom boxes*. Letting go of healthy guilt's pain, we keep the deepened self-knowledge, compassion, empathy, and spiritual growth.

Whereas healthy guilt opens the way to increasing our self-awareness, resolving our difficulties, improving our relationships, and growing spiritually, unhealthy guilt keeps us stuck in a continual restatement of our presumed unworthiness. Unhealthy guilt is unproductive and toxic to our peace of mind, wisdom, and ability to care for ourselves and others. In the state of unhealthy guilt, it is not the omission or commission of a specific act that triggers remorse. Instead, we live in a constant state of diminishment regardless of what we do or don't do. This painful state of being in which we feel defective, phoney, flawed, or unworthy is called shame. *People whose personalities are based on hiding these painful feelings of shame from themselves and others live in a state of unhealthy guilt.* They blame themselves for things that are not their fault, their responsibility, or even their business. Later in the chapter, there is a checklist of twenty-one thoughts, behaviors, and emotions that are characteristic of unhealthy guilt. But before we review these characteristics, we need to take a close look at the core emotion out of which both healthy and unhealthy guilt arise—shame.

SHAME AS AN INNATE RESPONSE (HEALTHY SHAME)

All of us can remember being ashamed about incidents in our lives. This one happened when I was fourteen. Standing at the bus stop outside the high school, I felt a sudden pop. The inexorable slithering of nylon against flesh turned me beet red. I stood paralyzed with fear. My undies were sliding down my leg toward an appointment with destiny. I was about to be revealed as suddenly different, unworthy, low. A loser, a nerd, a jerk. For two or three hideous minutes that seemed to stretch into eternity, I fantasized about being the butt of jokes and the subject of a hundred snickering phone calls and locker room conversations. Mercifully, I was saved by my knobby knees and long skirt. Hobbling to safety behind a bush, I pretended to check my books, and find one missing. I retreated into the school before I was discovered.

Shame feels like a sudden severing of our connection with the world. It leaves us feeling emotionally (if not literally) naked and revealed as something other than what we thought we were. Shame is shockingly painful and isolating. It breaks the bridges that bond us to others and leaves us feeling vulnerable and alone. Since the feeling of bondedness, of belonging and connectedness with others, is basic to our sense of self, shame temporarily destroys the sense of self. It is a powerful emotion. Indeed shame has been called the "master emotion," because childhood experiences of shame have the power to determine how we experience other emotions for the rest of our lives.

Shame is innate. We don't need to learn how to be ashamed. It is "factory installed," like the fight-or-flight response or the relaxation response. In shame, we suddenly catch and hold our breath. Eyes are downcast and the head is lowered. We are temporarily immobile. There is paralysis of action rather than the attempt to fight or flee. Instead of blood flowing to muscles, it rushes to the skin and we blush, often revealing our vulnerability against our will. Shame is the absolute picture of helplessness. We are beaten and we know it. In thinking about why such a powerful physiological reflex occurs, it is interesting to speculate on its survival value. Of what benefit is immobility and helplessness to social beings? Why would we evolve a mechanism to advertise the concession of defeat?

Human beings are social creatures. We are pack animals by nature. If you've ever owned a dog, you know quite a bit about the instinctive behavior of a pack animal. For example, when you yell at Fido for chewing the cord to the refrigerator, he looks submissive and ashamed, doesn't he? He lowers his head, crawls on his belly, beats his tail abjectly against the floor, and begs for mercy with his big brown eyes. You are the "top dog" in his pack, and his inherent ability to feel shame when he oversteps his boundaries and intrudes on your territory leads to ritual submissive behavior that calls off attack and favors survival. When Myrin and I were first married, one of our neighbors was a police officer who owned an attack-trained German shepherd. Our neighbor explained that standing completely still would prevent the dog from attacking, since immobility is a message of submission. You are no longer perceived as a threat when you stop moving.

While an analogy between human beings and dogs is necessarily oversimplified, I do believe that shame has survival value in the human social hierarchy as well. I once saw a little boy of about three at the supermarket with his father. The child was leaning out of the cart, grabbing at the different brightly colored boxes, as toddlers do. His father responded with such an outburst of anger and verbal abuse that I was terrified. Even though we were in a public place, it seemed certain that he would hit the child. But in response to the tirade, the little boy hung his head in shame, sitting in the cart like a meek little statue. The father looked at him for a minute, then continued down the aisle. It may be that an abuser finds it more difficult to hurt a submissive victim. There is relative safety in surrender.

In addition to a basic survival value, shame also has a higher-order social value. It is a core component of the painful remorse that accompanies healthy guilt. It signals our recognition that we have violated societal standards and is therefore critical to the development of conscience. In his comprehensive and thoughtful book *Healing the Shame That Binds You*, John Bradshaw notes that shame is present in infancy, while guilt emerges later in human development. We do not internalize societal ideas about right and wrong into a fledgling moral code of our own until we pass the age of three. According to personality theorist Erik Erikson, the three-year-old must then come to terms with opposing desires. On the other hand, the child wants his own way. On the other hand, he wants to honor the societal mores he has internalized.

If this stage of psychosocial development is properly completed, the child becomes "socialized to the pack" and understands that his own wants are secondary to a greater good. He has learned to experience healthy guilt. The proper development of healthy guilt requires two conditions: an internalized moral code and the capacity to feel shame that sounds an alarm when that code is violated. If the child does not learn to feel healthy guilt, he fails to develop conscience, a condition that is called sociopathy or psychopathy. Either moral codes are not properly internalized or the sense of shame is somehow lacking or suppressed. This is the unfortunate case with many criminals who hurt others without compunction.

SHAME AS A FALSE IDENTITY (UNHEALTHY SHAME)

While the capacity to feel shame is normal, adaptive, and a requirement for the development of healthy guilt, conscience, compassion, and empathy, it can take on a life of its own that is unrelated to its primary function as an alarm for overstepping boundaries. In Gershen Kaufman's scholarly and gentle book *Shame: The Power of Caring*, he distinguishes between shame as a passing emotion, a normal reaction to any sudden, unexpected exposure where we lose face, and shame as an identity, a state in which we feel alienated, deficient, despairing, and helpless in general, rather than as a reaction to a specific event.

> Contained in the experience of shame is the piercing awareness of ourselves as fundamentally deficient in some vital way as a human being. To live with shame is to experience the very essence or heart of the self as wanting. Shame is an impotence-making experience because it feels as though there is no way to relieve the matter, no way to restore the balance of things. *One has simply failed as a human being.* No single action is seen as wrong and, hence, reparable [p. 8, italics added].

Shame as an identity—what John Bradshaw calls *toxic shame*—means that we have lost our true identity and value as a human being. Out of touch with our worthiness, we fall prey to the sense of mistaken identity discussed in the last chapter. We see ourselves as flawed, as inferior. Self-esteem is dangerously low. Bradshaw links the case of mistaken identity to a false belief system based on shame. "I am flawed and defective as a human being. I am a mistake." This shame-based identity in turn gives rise to distorted thinking: "No one could love me as I am. I need something outside myself in order to be whole and okay."

Bradshaw traces how this distorted thinking leads to a whole range of addictive behaviors. Whether we choose to alter our mood and recover a temporary sense of power and connectedness through alcohol, drugs, sex, work, perfectionism, dependent or controlling relationships, or even some forms of religious belief and practice, we are really seeking the same thing: self-respect and a connectedness to a larger frame of meaning. We are searching both for our temporal self as a human being of unique worth and our eternal Self as part of a greater whole.

It is no mistake that purely psychologically based programs are relatively ineffective in dealing with addiction. Addictive behavior and the shame-based identity that underlies it are symptoms of what both William James and Gershen Kaufman call soul sickness. The cure for soul sickness requires psychological self-awareness and behavior change, but it goes beyond those goals to a reconnection with the Spirit, the Source of our being, which corrects the case of mistaken identity at its deepest level. This is why twelve-step programs, offered by Alcoholics Anonymous and other groups that are spiritually based as well as psychologically sophisticated, are such a potent force for healing shame and addiction.

SHAME AND SPIRITUALITY

We defined spirituality as a reconnection or, more correctly, a remembrance of our eternal connection with a lifeforce or power that we are part of. We "live and move and have our being" in that greater medium in much the way that a wave is part of the ocean. It is within us and also beyond us. Through it we are connected to all things and to a rich source of wisdom that we access in moments of inspiration and intuition. In those moments, the mind calms down and we center in the inner Self. In that remembrance, we become vividly aware that the lifeforce is the emotional energy we describe as love. In that remembrance, we are deeply aware of our own worthiness. We feel loving-kindness toward ourselves and others. Spiritual connection is the polar opposite of the isolated, unworthy feeling of unhealthy shame.

The need to recollect the spirit is a strong desire in all of us, although we may not recognize spiritual longing as such. The desire for love, peace, beauty, wisdom, and creativity are traditional spiritual longings. Addictive desires for achievement, power, recognition, and material goods that may make us lovable, acceptable, or at least invincible, thus soothing the inner shame, are also motivated by the spiritual longing for love.

The problem is that addictive behaviors reinforce our "false self," that set of fear-based personality traits and behaviors that we adopt in hopes of looking good to others or at least dulling the pain of our imagined unworthiness. The more we identify with the false self, known by different theorists as the "mask" or "as-if" personality, the more we stay separated from the true Self and from an understanding of the life experiences we have stored up within our souls. Shame literally makes us strangers to ourselves.

Dr. Charles Whitfield presents the following list of characteristics of the Real Self, as opposed to the false or shame-based self, in his excellent book *Healing the Child Within*.

Whitfield expands on his distinction between the Real Self and the false self as follows:

> Our Real Self is spontaneous, expansive, loving, giving, and communicating. Our True Self accepts ourselves and others. It feels, whether the feelings may be joyful or painful. And it expresses those feelings. Our Real Self accepts our feelings without judgment and fear, and allows them to exist as a valid way of assessing and appreciating life's events. . . . It can be childlike in the highest, most mature, and evolved sense of the word. It needs to play and to have fun. And yet it is vulnerable, perhaps because it is so open and trusting. It surrenders to itself, to others and ultimately to the universe. And yet it is powerful in the true sense of power. It is healthily self-indulgent, taking pleasure in receiving and being nurtured. It is also open to that vast and mysterious part of ourselves we call our unconscious. It pays attention to the messages that we receive daily from the unconscious, such as dreams, struggles and illness. By being real, it is free to grow. And while our co-dependent [false] self forgets, our Real Self remembers our Oneness with others and the universe [pp. 10, 11].

KNOW THYSELF

The spiritual search for meaning, wisdom, connectedness, and love begins with self-knowledge. We need to understand the false self and its basis in shame before we can let go of the fear that sustains it and begin to reorganize our personalities around the true Self. This is what we will do together in the next chapter. The Catch-22 of the shame-based personality, however, is that we are too ashamed of ourselves to engage in

Real Self	*False Self**
Authentic self	Unauthentic self, mask
True self	False self, persona
Genuine	Ungenuine, "as-if" personality
Spontaneous	Plans and plods
Expansive, loving	Contracting, fearful
Giving, communicating	Withholding
Accepting of self and others	Envious, critical, idealized, perfectionistic
Compassionate	Other-oriented, overly conforming
Loves unconditionally	Loves conditionally
Feels feelings, including appropriate, spontaneous, current anger	Denies or hides feelings, including long-held anger (resentment)
Assertive	Aggressive and/or passive
Intuitive	Rational, logical
Child within, inner child/ability to be childlike	Overdeveloped parent/adult scripts/ may be childish
Needs to play and have fun	Avoids play and fun
Vulnerable	Pretends always to be strong
Powerful in true sense	Limited power
Trusting	Distrusting
Enjoys being nurtured	Avoids being nurtured
Surrenders	Controls, withdraws
Self-indulgent	Self-righteous
Open to the unconscious	Blocks unconscious material
Remembers our oneness	Forgets our oneness/feels separate
Free to grow	Tends to act out unconscious, often painful patterns repeatedly
Private self	Public self

*Dr. Whitfield titles this column "co-dependent self," a term we will define later in the section on Unhealthy Guilt and Adult Children of Alcoholics.

honest introspection! Knowing oneself would mean admitting the normal weaknesses and fears that every human being has, but a shame-based person tries to hide these from himself out of shame.

> A shame-based person will guard against exposing his inner self to others, but more significantly, he will guard against exposing himself to himself. Toxic shame is so excruciating because it is the painful exposure of the believed failure of self to self. In toxic shame the self becomes an object that can't be trusted. As an object that can't be trusted, one experiences oneself as untrustworthy.
>
> —John Bradshaw, *Healing the Shame That Binds You* [p. 10]

The age-old advice, "Know thyself," is hard to follow when shame gets in the way of self-honesty, yet psychological and spiritual traditions agree that self-awareness is the road to recovery from soul sickness. Knowing ourselves means accepting ourselves just as we are, without getting hung up on looking good. How many of us deny certain emotions like anger because we think that "nice" people don't get angry? Anger, like any emotion, is neither good nor bad. It just is. Emotions are messages about the world, and repressing them simply keeps us in ignorance. It doesn't qualify us for sainthood.

Not until I had suffered for many years and come to the point where my lack of self-awareness and thus self-knowledge had crippled me with illness, poor relationships, anxiety, depression, panic, and perfectionism did I finally surrender and face the inner pain of shame. It was not, and is not, easy to peel away the layers of protective self-deceit that form around shame and give rise to the behavior pattern of unhealthy guilt. It is still sometimes easier for me to lose myself in work or reading than to face painful feelings that are tapping on my shoulder, trying to give me a message about my past and its relation to present behaviors and relationships. It is still sometimes easier to pretend things are fine when they are not, to do things I don't want to do because it is hard to say no, to offer myself up as a victim rather than speaking my mind—to give away my power. But I have learned that the consequences of these forms of self-deceit are disastrous. They make the moment more comfortable and the future much more difficult.

The first step in my own ongoing recovery from unhealthy guilt and the shame that underlies it was recognition of its symptoms. How does unhealthy guilt distort our thoughts, emotions, and behaviors? Over the years, I have compiled a list of twenty-one thoughts, emotions, and behaviors that accompany a shame-based identity and yield a working definition of the unhealthy guilt that shame creates. Admitting how we feel, without getting down on ourselves for feeling that way, is how we learn to listen to emotional messages, free ourselves from the past, and start our psychospiritual healing.

As you read through the following characteristics of unhealthy guilt, be gentle with yourself as you begin to own the ones that ring a bell for you. Recognizing these in yourself is not an invitation to self-criticism and more guilt. It is an invitation to self-awareness and the reconnection with love and free choice that it affords us. In the interest of making it easier to look at ourselves, I've compiled the list with a sense of humor so that we won't get bogged down in guilt's tendency to make us take ourselves too seriously.

TWENTY-ONE EXPRESSIONS OF UNHEALTHY GUILT

1. I'm Overcommitted

Taking on more than any human being can reasonably accomplish is a common characteristic of unhealthy guilt. Too many projects, too much to do, never enough time. This habit, a major cause of stress, is fed by the difficulty we have in saying no—both to our own needs to achieve and to other people's expectations of us. Overcommitment is based on the illusion that we can recapture our love, and that of others, by collecting achievements that prove our worth. Furthermore, overcommitment is an addiction that keeps us anesthetized to the anxious, empty feelings that will inevitably surface if we are left alone without distractions. Overcommitment is a way of avoiding our pain. It blocks the process of recovery.

2. I Really Know How to Worry

It's midnight. Your daughter had an 11:30 curfew, but she isn't home yet. The movie could have gotten out late, or maybe she's having a good time and forgot to check the clock. Maybe she's even being an adolescent and testing your limits a little. But the most probable explanation is that she has been raped, kidnapped, killed, or at least permanently maimed in a car crash. Breathing heavily, you decide to be reasonable and wait until 12:15 before calling the police and all the local emergency rooms.

The immediate escalation of any event into a world-class catastrophe is what psychologist Albert Ellis calls *awfulizing*. Its most amazing feature is that little or no objective evidence is required to come to conclusions of unprecedented gloom and doom. This kind of worry is the outer projection of our innermost fear—that of our own destruction. For, without the knowledge of love, fear is all that remains, and we can never feel safe.

3. I'm a Compulsive Helper

The ranks of helping professionals—nurses, therapists, volunteer committee chairpersons—are bulging with the guilty. Several years ago, earlier in my own ongoing healing, a friend called me a professional saviorette. It made me mad at the time, but he was absolutely right. But you don't have to be a helping professional to be a professional helper who feels that it is your responsibility to fix everyone else's problems. In reaching out to others, we naturally try to give them the love we so desperately need ourselves, but since we don't know how to love ourselves, attempts to love and save others often backfire. Compulsive helping is not an authentic reaching out to another person's Self from our own. Instead, it is the reaching out of a fearful part of ourself to a fearful part of someone else. This process is like the blind leading the blind—both are likely to fall into a ditch.

4. I'm Always Apologizing for Myself

When canceling your dentist appointment turns into a five-minute explanation of how sick your mother-in-law is and how there is no one to help her, and that you are desperately sorry for the inconvenience you have caused and that you will do everything in your power to make sure that you never repeat such a heinous crime again, you are in trouble. Feeling that everyone else is the judge and jury of our souls, we apologize continually, often making ourselves downright obnoxious. Nothing we do is ever quite good enough. The present we chose isn't exactly right, so we tell Aunt Sue how to exchange it before she can even get the wrappings off. The house isn't clean enough, we didn't really mean to say that, the chicken we cooked for dinner is too dry. And we're sorry, *so* sorry, really.

5. I Often Wake Up Feeling Anxious or Have Periods When I Am Anxious for Days or Weeks

If we're lucky, the anxiety begins after a good night's sleep. If not, it happens in the middle of the night or awakens us early, and the mental wheels start to spin. Ruminations over the past take on a life of their own, "*If only* I had or hadn't done this or that," accompanied by worry over future uncertainties, "*What if* this or that happens?" We worry about all the things that we might have done wrong already or might do wrong soon. If we are overcommitted, we worry about how we can fit everything in and who will be angry with us when we can't meet our commitment in time. Our anxiety often masks anger as well. After all, those people we are saving, helping, or demonstrating our achievements to begin to look like our persecutors sometimes, don't they?

6. I'm Always Blaming Myself

If your daughter fails algebra, it's *your* fault, because whatever you did or didn't do as her parent just wasn't good enough. If you lose your job because there's a recession and engineers are getting laid off, it's never bad luck or a sign of the times. And it is never, *never* an opportunity. It is a terrible thing, and it is all your fault because you are stupid, lazy, a jerk, a loser, or suffer from some other fatal flaw that is central to your constant self-criticism. This kind of pessimistic thinking is a hallmark of unhealthy guilt and continuously reinforces the helplessness so central to shame as an identity.

7. I Worry About What Other People Think of Me

We may lie in bed and rerun conversations. We said the wrong thing *again*. That person is probably lying awake right now thinking about how insensitive, stupid, or naive we are. Just thinking about it makes us feel ashamed, even though everything seemed okay at the time of the conversation. Or perhaps we have just finished a big project and feel pretty good about it. If the feedback we get is positive, we are elated. But, if there is any negative feedback, even though it will improve the project tremendously, all our good feelings evaporate. We don't hear feedback as a dialogue about ideas, we hear it as an indictment of self. We are a failure. This is called *attachment to praise and blame*. It means we have granted other people the power to determine our state of worth. It means we are helpless.

8. I Hate It When People Are Angry with Me

Our antennae are always sniffing the air for anger. The boss is quiet and preoccupied this week. With no objective evidence, we may deduce that she is angry at us. We forget to call back a friend when we said we would, and then we feel so guilty that we keep procrastinating. We are afraid that she will be angry with us, so we withdraw, making a bad situation out of an oversight. When someone actually confronts us with anger, we feel so vulnerable and overwhelmed that we will do almost anything to get off the hook and restore ourself to their good graces, including lying, cheating, and compromising our ethics. Nothing is as important as survival, and anger seems like a direct threat to it. As tiny children, we believed that our survival depended on being lovable, and deep down inside, the frightened child within still believes that the angry person holds the power of life and death over her.

9. I'm Not As Good As People Think I Am. I Just Have Everybody Fooled

Someday people are going to find out that we really don't know as much, do as much, care as much, love as much, as they think. We are actually frauds. Only circumstances have dictated that we have come as far as we have. Most other people in our boots are actually much smarter and more competent than we are. Psychologists call this the *imposter syndrome*, and it afflicts many competent and bright people who define their worth in terms of what they can produce rather than who they are, what John Bradshaw calls acting like a *human doing* rather than a *human being*. In fact, the problem is that we don't really know who we are, and so we feel empty and confused.

10. I'm a Doormat

We try so hard to be good that we are often the one to take on the extra project. We do twice as much work around the house, the office, the school cookout as co-workers, family, or friends. Furthermore, even if it's someone else's job, we often jump in and do it before they've got a chance! This pattern inevitably leads to anger because it forces other people into the role of "aggressor," since we insist on being the "victim" of their fantasied insensitivity toward us. In family situations, "doormatting" creates the famous *martyr complex*, which is guaranteed to make us vastly unpopular in spite of all our efforts. After all, few people care to play the role of the ungrateful, lazy, ne'er-do-well that the martyr needs for self-definition.

11. I Never Have Any Time for Myself

How could you? Unhealthy guilt keeps us too busy working, helping, saving the world, emptying the dishwasher, and worrying about all the other things for which there is no time. We are always the last priority on our own list. Even though we know that exercise, meditation, or plain old rest make us feel better, something else is always more pressing. The needs of others always take precedence over our own needs, reflecting the low self-esteem that accompanies shame as an identity. When we don't take time to restore ourselves—in spirit as well as in body—we reinforce the sense of isolation and helplessness that underlies unhealthy guilt. If there's no time to walk the beach or watch a sunset, if there's no time to listen to our hearts, we're not really living. And we're not really happy.

12. I Worry That Other People Are Better Than I Am

When I was first learning to cut ultrathin sections of specimens to view under the electron microscope, I was in a hurry to do it perfectly. There were many steps, including breaking knives from huge sheets of glass, bonding a waterfilled "boat" to the knife in order to float off the sections, and then learning to approach the specimen slowly with a big, complicated apparatus know as a microtome. My professor made short work of this and could get great sections in no time. I was jealous of the ease with which he worked, and I complained to him about how slow I was. His response really surprised me. "How egotistical can you get?" he bridled. "I've been doing this for twelve years, and you expect to be as good in a week!" In guilty thinking, success and failure is a constant theme, breeding envy and competitiveness.

13. "Must" and "Should" Are My Favorite Words

Perhaps you are sitting in the living room, unwinding in front of the TV. Although you are enjoying watching the news, suddenly you remember those two phone calls you should make. Without even thinking, you bolt out of the chair and pick up the phone, again putting someone else's needs before your own. Or perhaps you have invited friends for dinner. All afternoon you compulsively clean and cook, making more than anyone wants to eat anyway. When the company comes, you would enjoy relaxing and talking with the group, but you must get back to the kitchen and oversee the banquet. No wonder you feel stressed and anxious rather than comfortable and calm. Musts and shoulds are a great way to motivate yourself as a human *doing*, but they block the joy of human *being*.

14. I Can't Stand Criticism

Even garden variety questions are often perceived as critical assaults that require immediate self-protection. As in, "Gee, dear, did you get around to calling the roofer today?" "Call the roofer? How could I? After all, I've been on the go since 7:30 this morning. I didn't get out of work until almost 6:00—it was so busy that there wasn't a minute to make a call. I'm completely exhausted. I didn't even have time for lunch. On top of it all, we were out of milk, bread, eggs, and cat food. I had to go to the market on the way home. You know how busy I am." Since an answer of this kind sounds like an accusation (how could he even ask when he knows how busy you are), your spouse is now angry at you. Self-defense against reproach is what we think protects us from the rejection and abandonment that we fear so much. Tragically, our defense consists in dishing out the same rejection that we fear, so no one wins.

15. I'm a Perfectionist

You take an exam and get 90 percent. Are you happy? Not if you're a perfectionist. Instead of taking joy in the 90 percent they get, perfectionists would rather complain about the 10 percent they missed. Statistically, it is a fact that no one can do "their best" 100 percent of the time. Half the time we do better than our average, and half the time we do worse. That's statistical perfection as defined by the laws of probability. It takes a lot of nerve to believe that we can or should be able to outwit natural laws, but perfectionism requires just that. As a strategy that evolved to ensure love and approval, it is rooted deep in the fears and longings of childhood, making it an emotional need, not an intellectual choice. Perfectionism makes no sense at all from a rational perspective and can be corrected only by returning to its roots in childhood, as we will do together in the next chapter.

16. I Worry About Being Selfish

Even though you dedicate so much time to helping other people, you secretly worry that you might be selfish. The reason for this is simple. You are often angry at the very people you are bending over backward to assist, because helping them leaves so little time and energy for you. Instead of acknowledging your anger as a signal that things are out of balance, you interpret it as an inappropriate feeling that you should not have. After all, any really good human being would happily continue giving, oblivious to their own needs, until they dropped on the floor in a heap, wouldn't they? Isn't this true greatness? A good friend once reminded me that even Mother Teresa has the Sisters of Mercy to help her! Acknowledging your own needs first will allow you to help others when *they* need it, not when *you* need it. This is sanity, not selfishness.

17. I Hate to Take Any Assistance or Ask for Help

Perhaps you are standing in an elevator with both hands full. Instead of asking someone to push the button for you, you press it with your nose. Your in-laws are visiting for a week. Instead of asking them to share the cooking and cleaning (which would make them much more comfortable), you run around trying to do everything yourself. By the end of the week, you're exhausted and angry, right? Most guilty people find that it's much easier to give than to receive, and that it's almost impossible to receive if it requires asking.

Yet giving and receiving are really the battery poles between which love flows, aren't they? So refusing to receive is not an act of generosity at all; it's a subtle kind of selfishness that dams up the flow of love and keeps us separate from the Spirit.

18. I Can't Take Compliments

"Wow, Ellen, what a great dress!" "Oh, it's just a hand-me-down from my sister-in-law. She really has great taste in clothes." Is this familiar? The guilty response to compliments is a fascinating paradox. On the one hand, we yearn to be perfect and thrive on approval. But when it's freely given, we push it away, focusing instead on possible imperfections that might invalidate the compliment. For example, you bought the dress in a bargain basement, and it's really not as special as it looks. You bought it at Saks, and you're embarrassed by how much money you spent. You bought it in blue, which is not your best color. It is too dressy for the occasion. It is too plain for the occasion. It is just right for the occasion, but it is wrong for the weather, which suddenly changed. You gained five pounds, and the waistband is killing you. You lost five pounds, and it doesn't show off your figure. You have lousy taste anyhow, and the compliment was a lie. Remember our suitcase for guilt? You need a matching piece just to pack your clothes guilt in!

19. I Sometimes Worry That I Am Being—or Will Be—Punished for My Sins

When something bad happens, the psychological pessimist always blames herself. Psychologist Martin Seligman describes pessimist as the self-critical, helpless, and hopeless attitude of "It's all my fault. I mess up everything I do, and it's the story of my life." The spiritual pessimist takes it a step further. "It's all my fault, and this bad thing is happening because God is punishing me for my sins." As we'll discuss in Chapter Seven, psychological pessimism favors the adoption of fear-based beliefs in a judgmental, punitive God. Spiritual pessimism saps our strength and keeps us prisoners of fear, helplessness, and guilt. It is the antithesis of spiritual optimism, which is based on the inner "knowing" of God as love, and the corresponding faith that life's bad events are occasions for soul growth, not punishments for unworthiness.

20. I Worry About My Body a Lot

Guilty people are prone to both illness and hypochondria. Seventy-five percent of doctor's visits are attributed to stress-related disorders, including fatigue, muscle tension, gastrointestinal and cardiovascular disorders, increased susceptibility to infection, allergy, and depressed immunity. Guilty people also tend to awfulize about aches and pains, like the backache that started last Monday. It could have been the flat tire you fixed, the picture you hung, or even the encroaching signs of middle age. But most likely it's cancer. Your number is up. You are certain. But if the backache goes away, don't worry. Tomorrow, or a week from tomorrow, you may feel dizzy. This could be stress, an ear infection, or maybe even multiple sclerosis. However, after due deliberation you decide a brain tumor is the likeliest explanation! Worrying about the body deflects attention from emotional self-awareness. It's one more way of numbing the pain of inner shame.

And last, but certainly not least:

21. I Can't Say No

This little word fills the guilty with fear. Since we so desperately need approval, saying no is a terrible risk. Someone might think we are bad or selfish. Someone might even feel put off or angry with us. Since we are not entitled to have any space or to need anything other than the opportunity to help others, why bother saying no? There's nothing in it for us but anxiety and rejection.

UNHEALTHY GUILT AND ADULT CHILDREN OF ALCOHOLICS

During the years over which I compiled this list, I started to familiarize myself with some of the literature on adult children of alcoholics. Adult children of alcoholics frequently grow up with shame-based personalities and become what the addiction community terms codependents. The word "codependent" comes from the observation that even though the adult child of an alcoholic may not become an alcoholic, he or she will usually choose relationships with people who have addictions to a substance like alcohol or drugs, to some process like work, or even to religious fanaticism. There is a nearly unerring, unconscious radar that zeros in on relationships that repeat our childhood experiences. Adult children thus become codependent on the addictions of significant others to continue their familiar way of relating to the world. In fact, codependents are also addicts. They are addicted to guilt.

I was struck by the overlap in the characteristics of unhealthy guilt and the characteristics of adult children of alcoholics that have been widely circulated. Below, you can read a list of fourteen such items compiled in the mid-1970s by Tony A., a member of Alcoholics Anonymous, which was published in Dennis Wholey's book for adult children *Becoming Your Own Parent*. The list was generated from Tony A.'s personal inventory of himself, called fourth-step work—a searching psychological and moral inventory designed to increase self-awareness.

While Tony A.'s list reflects his childhood in an alcoholic home, we're all adult children of somebody. Charles Whitfield estimates that between 80 and 95 percent of all adults grew up in some sort of dysfunctional family where they developed a shame-based identity similar to adult children of alcoholics. Because of this, many people who did not grow up in alcoholic homes nonetheless feel a tingle of recognition when they read a list of characteristics of adult children of alcoholics. This list can apply just as well to children of self-centered parents, workaholics, parents absent from the home because of economic necessity, physically ill parents, mentally ill parents, sexually, emotionally, or spiritually abusive parents, and smothering parents who did everything for their children except let them become themselves. Because of these similarities, people whose parents were not alcoholic frequently find considerable benefit in attending Alanon or Adult Children of Alcoholics programs and working the twelve steps to recovery that could profit the majority of us.

This is Tony A.'s list:

1. We became isolated and afraid of people and authority figures.

2. We became approval seekers and lost our identity in the process.

3. We are frightened by angry people and any personal criticism.

4. We either become alcoholics, marry them—or both—or find another compulsive personality, such as a workaholic, to fulfill our sick abandonment needs.

5. We live life from the viewpoint of victims and are attracted by that weakness in our love and friendship relationships.

6. We have an overdeveloped sense of responsibility; it is easier for us to be concerned with others rather than ourselves; this enables us not to look too closely at our faults.

7. We get guilt feelings when we stand up for ourselves instead of giving in to others.

8. We become addicted to excitement.

9. We confuse love and pity, and tend to "love" people we can "pity" and "rescue."

10. We have "stuffed" our feelings from our traumatic childhoods and have lost the ability to feel or express our feelings, because it hurts so much.

11. We judge ourselves harshly and have a very low sense of self-esteem.

12. We are dependent personalities who are terrified of abandonment, and we will do anything to hold onto a relationship in order not to experience the painful abandonment feelings that we received from living with sick people who were never there emotionally for us.

13. Alcoholism is a family disease, and we became para-alcoholics who took on the characteristics of that disease, even though we did not pick up the drink.

14. Para-alcoholics are reactors rather than actors.

Para-alcoholics are innocent bystanders damaged by alcoholic behavior and trained in the distorted thinking that underlies addiction. In nonalcoholic homes, we could call such children para*shame*oholics. There are many of us. We'll read some of our stories and reflect on how the distorted thinking that we call unhealthy guilt began, in the next chapter. Here I would like to examine the characteristic shared by all children raised in shame—low self-esteem.

SHAME AND SELF-ESTEEM

Psychologist Nathaniel Branden calls self-esteem the reputation we have with ourselves. When we live our lives out of shame and believe that we are unworthy, that reputation is low—and low self-esteem is the result. Our relationship to ourself is strained and burdensome. In *Honoring the Self*, Branden reminds us:

> We stand in the midst of an almost infinite network of relationships: to other people, to things, to the universe. And yet, at three o'clock in the morning, when we are alone with ourselves, we are aware that the most intimate and powerful of all relationships and the one we can never escape is the relationship to ourselves. No significant aspect of our thinking, motivation, feelings, or behavior is unaffected by our self-evaluation. We are organisms who are not only conscious but self-conscious. That is our glory and, at times, our burden [p. 1].

While human beings are intrinsically self-conscious—capable of self-awareness—a primary side effect of shame is constriction of our self-awareness. Because the deep sense of inadequacy that accompanies shame is too much to consciously bear, we develop psychological defense mechanisms to protect ourselves from our own self-criticism and self-destructive judgmentalness. For example, since our own anger is often too frightening to admit, we tend to project it outside of ourselves and see other people as angry, or as blaming, aggressive, unfair, judgmental, controlling, or mean. In thinking of ourselves as the victims of others, we can disown the reality that we are actually victims of ourselves. The more we insist on not being aware, the more trapped we become.

The recovery from unhealthy guilt and the shame and low self-esteem on which it rests begins with the willingness to be self-aware, to be honest about our thoughts and feelings, as we'll discuss in depth in the chapters to come. Branden summarizes the skills of awareness that we must be willing to practice in recovering from low self-esteem—what he calls learning to *honor the self*—as follows:

> The first act of honoring the self is the asserting of consciousness: the choice to think, to be aware, to send the searchlight of consciousness outward toward the world and inward toward our own being. To default on this effort is to default on the self at the most basic level.
>
> To honor the self is to be willing to think independently, to live by our own mind, and to have the courage of our own perceptions and judgments.
>
> To honor the self is to be willing to know not only what we think but also what we feel, what we want, need, desire, suffer over, are frightened or angered by—and to accept our right to experience such feelings. The opposite of this attitude is denial, disowning, repression—self-repudiation.
>
> To honor the self is to preserve an attitude of self-acceptance—

which means to accept what we are, without self-oppression or self-castigation, without any pretense about the truth of our own being, pretense aimed at deceiving either ourselves or anyone else.

To honor the self is to live authentically, to speak and act from our innermost convictions and feelings.

To honor the self is to refuse to accept unearned guilt and to do our best to correct such guilt as we may have earned.

To honor the self is to be committed to our right to exist, which proceeds from the knowledge that our life does not belong to others and that we are not here on earth to live up to someone else's expectations. To many people, this is a terrifying responsibility.

To honor the self is to be in love with our own life, in love with our own possibilities for growth and experiencing joy, in love with the process of discovering and exploring our distinctively human potentialities [pp. 3, 4].

OVERCOMING THE TYRANNY OF BLACK-AND-WHITE THINKING

Underlying all the distorted thinking that follows from forgetting our true identity as beings of love, worth, and wisdom is the fear of being bad, which, in turn, might lead to rejection and abandonment. In a child's mind, rejection and abandonment are equivalent to death. This deep fear sets up a rigid mental censor, a psychological defense mechanism, that splits our thoughts, emotions, and behaviors into two mutually exclusive categories—good or bad, black or white, safe or unsafe. Splitting means we're either perfect or a failure, a saint or a sinner, and these are categories that we apply just as rigidly to other people. The self-criticism, self-deceit, and loss of self-awareness that accompany splitting keep us helpless, powerless, ashamed, enraged, and anxious—a steep price for appearing to be "good."

Rooting out the characteristics of unhealthy guilt rests on the ability to accept the range of grays that make us human. No one is all black or all white. We are each a composite, a mosaic of different thoughts, emotions, and choices of behavior. Each of us is more mature in some areas than in others. This doesn't make us "bad"—it just means that we have certain "growing edges." *Rather than thinking in terms of good and bad, it is more helpful to think in terms of conscious and unconscious, aware and unaware.* The more aware we are, the further along the road to recovery from guilt we will progress. For example, repressing anger to appear virtuous and stay safe is typical of the false self's constriction of self-awareness. It is unconscious and habitual. In the same way, an angry outburst whose effect on self and others is ill-considered is similarly unconscious. In contrast, recognizing one's anger, feeling okay about having it, and then expressing it in a way that is not hurtful to self or others is a conscious choice.

I know a Buddhist meditation teacher. He is kind, wise, compassionate, *and* he smokes cigarettes. It is his choice to do so. Those who self-righteously believe that such beings should be pure as Ivory Flakes in every habit of the flesh will miss a wonderful teacher. It is likewise possible to be a fine parent *and* lose your temper once in a while. We can be kind *and* selfish, loving *and* occasionally judgmental, a nice person *and* very angry at the moment. And no matter who we are and how hard we have worked to become whole and aware, we will still make mistakes. If we can accept our humanity with open-mindedness and awareness, rather than censoring ourselves out of shame, we will be more capable of choosing behaviors that maximize our freedom and happiness.

In rejecting the tyranny of black-and-white, "either/or" thinking, we become more flexible, interesting, playful, and humorous. We become less rigid, self-righteous, stuffy, judgmental, and constricted. Reflect on the words of this ancient poem, written in the voice of a female wisdom and buried in the Egyptian desert town of Nag Hammadi more than 1600 years ago. The poem was unearthed as part of a collection of fifty-two gnostic (from the Greek word for inner knowing) manuscripts in 1945. They date from the time of Christ:

For I am the first and the last.
I am the honored one and the scorned one.
I am the whore and the holy one.
I am the wife and the virgin . . .
I am the barren one
and many are her sons. . . .

For I am knowledge and ignorance.
I am shame and boldness.
I am shameless; I am ashamed.
I am strength and I am fear.
I am war and I am peace.

I am the one who is disgraced and the great one . . .
I am godless,
and I am the one whose God is great.

—Selected from
"The Thunder, Perfect Mind,"
in *The Nag Hammadi Library*,
James M. Robinson, Editor

SUGGESTIONS FOR THE READER

1. Which of the characteristics of unhealthy guilt, the false self, or adult children of alcoholics did you relate to?

2. Sit down with a journal at a time when you are willing to devote an hour or two to yourself. Write about your guilty characteristics. If possible, share your self-examination with a trusted friend or relative, or discuss it with a therapist.

3. Become aware of splitting. Notice and root out black-and-white or good-or-bad thinking. When you are caught in it, take a deep breath and back off. Ask yourself, "What am I unaware of? What am I really feeling?" Whether you are engaging in self-judgment or judging others, remember the gnostic poem. It is not "good" or "bad" that counts. All nature, including human nature, is made of opposites. It is awareness and self-acceptance that sets us free.

CHAPTER THREE

The Inner Child's Drama

Flying home to Boston from San Francisco on the "red eye," I was once aroused from a 6:00 A.M. torpor by the unexpected sound of laughter and delight. Two rows ahead, a toddler was playing a spirited game of peek-a-boo over the top of the seat with a man in his eighties. Their faces were shining, and in no time a knot of passengers gathered round, drawn to the joy like flowers opening to the sun. Tired strangers on a cramped airplane suddenly became fellow travelers on a more enduring journey. Bonded by shared smiles, tender looks, and eyes misted by the sudden gratitude for life that overflowed in unsuspecting hearts, we shared a moment of magic and meaning. The "Natural Child" within each of us momentarily awakened and shared in the delight.

Children are abundantly *enthusiastic*—a word whose root meaning in Greek is literally "possessed by God." Naturally present in the moment, children are given to spontaneously enjoying life as it happens. It's always a little frustrating for parents who buy toys for their toddlers to find that they may prefer the cellophane wrapping! Wouldn't it be great if adults could take such pleasure in little things again? This exuberant gratitude for life is what makes children so endearing despite all the trouble they are to care for! Little children approach life with what Rabbi Abraham Heschel calls "radical amazement." They are in tune with and entranced by the mystery of life that they embody. They are curious and receptive to its ever-changing flow of events.

As long as children feel loved, their joy is evident, even in the worst situations. I'll never forget my trepidation at seeing the slums of Bombay. The poverty was overwhelming and hygiene all but lacking. Nonetheless, the air was filled with the laughter of children at play. Psychiatrist Elisabeth Kübler-Ross speaks movingly of an even worse situation. Visiting a children's barracks in one of the German death camps after the war, she had expected to see evidence of terror. Instead the walls were covered with drawings of butterflies, an ancient symbol for the Spirit. The intrinsic ability of the human soul to flourish even in dire adversity is a tribute to the vitality of the Natural Child that remains within each of us, connected wordlessly to the Spirit, even as we grow old.

CONDITIONAL AND UNCONDITIONAL LOVE

Through the years of growing up, the Natural Child, the Real Self—the Divine core of our personality—gets hidden underneath a veil spun out of a collection of instructions on how we are supposed to act in order to be lovable. When our value is contingent on behaving and feeling in prescribed ways, we become victims of *conditional love*. Because love is such a potent reinforcer of behavior, we quickly learn to experience and express primarily those thoughts, emotions, and behaviors that are rewarded by love. As we'll see, we likewise learn to repress and deny those parts of ourselves that are shamed. Through this powerful conditioning, we lose the freedom to experience the world as it is happening. Instead, we experience the world through selective filters created by the extension and withdrawal of love. We come to see, as the apostle Paul said, "through a glass, darkly."

I have never seen the power of *unconditional love* more powerfully demonstrated than in a documentary film about Mother Teresa in which she is shown ministering to sick and dying children. When asked why she bothers to care for children who will soon die anyway, she replies simply that love is the birthright of every person. It's what we're all here on earth for. There's a particularly moving part in the film where Mother Teresa is caring for a severely spastic child who is dying of malnutrition. His wasted face and limbs are contorted in a twisted mask of pain and fear. Mother Teresa begins to "lay on hands" with great tenderness, smiling her love into the frightened eyes. Within minutes, the child's limbs have miraculously relaxed, and his face is full of peace and joy. The Natural Child in him, temporarily asleep, is reawakened by her love. Watching that sequence, I found it easy to see that unconditional love—given to us simply because we are—completes the circuit that connects us to life.

The need for love is, indeed, the most basic condition for survival. Without it, we will die in infancy. Children whose physical needs are provided for—they are fed and changed—but who are not touched and held, cooed at and responded to, literally stop growing. Their pituitary glands don't put out enough growth hormone, and they grow very slowly, if at all. This used to be a common occurrence in premature babies isolated in incubators. Now we know that when nurses and parents massage these tiny babies several times a day, they grow much faster and suffer fewer complications than when left alone in their aseptic environments.

This wasting away, called failure-to-thrive syndrome, is also endemic in foundling homes where care is given on schedule rather than in response to the needs of the child. Such children become depressed and withdrawn, antisocial and desperately afraid. After several months in such an environment, they withdraw into a joyless world of their own and often shriek in terror when approached. Many of them die as young children, and those who do survive are psychologically scarred. These poor children are sad scientific proof of what we all know in our hearts—that love is the lifeforce itself.

Fortunately, most of us got enough love to let our cells know we were alive, but many of us also got conditional messages. We came to believe that we were lovable when we acted in certain ways, but not in others. Perhaps we were lovable if we were quiet and didn't disturb mommy and daddy, did well in school, or excelled in sports. Some of us learned that we were lovable when we were happy, but not when we were sad or angry. Others of us learned that our worth depended on hiding some family secret—acting out a facade that hid addiction, sorrow, mental illness, or other pain, and made the family appear "normal."

THE INTERPERSONAL BRIDGE

Love is a reflection of mutuality in relationship. When a baby pulls her shirt up over her face, then whisks it down and starts to laugh in a game of peek-a-boo, most often the parent will start to laugh as well. The baby has engaged her parent, who then responds from a delighted frame of reference. As the game goes on, the two continue to create fresh frames of reference for one another. They play at curiosity, surprise, cat-and-mouse, responding to one another newly in each moment. They are in synch, tied together by a bond of mutuality, and love flows freely between them. They are present to one another. They trust the interaction to be caring, so they are open and creative. Although in this case one partner is a baby and one is an adult, they are relating to one another as Natural Child to Natural Child. Self to Self. Center to center. Joy to joy.

Psychiatrist Gershen Kaufman calls the bond of love and trust between two individuals the *interpersonal bridge*. It is the cornerstone of human interaction. When love is flowing across the bridge, we are in tune with our core, our center. We feel the delight of the moment. We bask in peace, love, joy, and trust because the natural light of the Self shines through. This is happiness, our fondest hope as human beings and the most basic reason for which all the activities of life are undertaken. Interpersonal bridges are the foundation for trust.

Trust is important to adults, but it is crucial to children because they have such a limited notion of how the world operates. Trust means that the world stays constant. If the sky is blue and clouds are white today, the child needs to know they will be the same colors tomorrow. If Mommy praises Molly for picking up her toys today, Molly assumes that picking them up will please Mommy tomorrow. If rules change in midstream, the child's tenuous picture of "reality" collapses, and she will hold herself to blame for the painful feelings of confusion and shame that follow. A toddler who has been delighting Mommy by picking up her dress and dancing around the living room with her undies exposed will be suddenly shocked and ashamed if she is angrily reprimanded for the same behavior in the supermarket.

At the moment of reprimand, the world stops working according to the rules. The interpersonal bridge is severed. Feeling scared and isolated, the child wonders what she did to bring this disaster about. Does it mean she will be abandoned? Does it mean that Mommy will stay angry forever? Does it mean that she will never be loved again? To a small child who knows so little about the world, a fragile being whose life is totally dependent on parental care, broken bridges are as frightening as death.

The emotional response to the sudden collapse of reality that follows broken bridges is shame. When love flowed across the bridge, we were connected and secure. When the love stopped flowing, we were isolated, helpless, and afraid. In shame, we are at the mercy of a powerful other on whom our survival seems to depend. As small children, no matter what happened to shame us we came to the conclusion that it was all our fault. We weren't good enough. The world collapsed *because of us*. No wonder early shaming creates the unhealthy need to control everything!

I once watched a mother picking her way through downtown traffic with a stroller in which her eight- or nine-month-old son was reclining. The child struggled to sit up and look around, finally grabbing onto the siderail of the stroller and pulling himself upright. He had a look of great delight and accomplishment on his face. But Mom was preoccupied with getting through the traffic and must have thought she could move faster if he was lying flat. She ignored his triumph and gave him a gentle shove onto his back. His eyes bugged out in sudden surprise. This is *not* how the world is supposed to work! He held his breath in shock and then began to whimper pitifully. Fortunately, Mom reconsidered the effect of her action. She stopped, picked up her son, comforted him, and restored the interpersonal bridge. Then she sat him up in the stroller and off they went.

That was a fortunate baby. Some of us had parents with problems—they were too busy, in turmoil as a result of their own childhood, alcoholic, ill, ignorant, or physically, emotionally, or spiritually abusive. They may have broken bridges quite often without noticing or caring, but in either case without stopping to repair them. And no matter how well-intentioned a parent may be, it is impossible to be completely tuned in to the needs of a child all the time. Every parent breaks bridges, sometimes in small ways and sometimes in more serious ways. Life is a patchwork of bridges made, broken, and hopefully mended. The ancient wisdom that we can grow strongest at our broken places gives a deeper significance to the wounds we all inevitably endure. Life's deepest learnings come when we take the opportunity to mend broken bridges, as we will discuss in Part Three when we explore forgiveness and relationships.

SHAME AND BROKEN BRIDGES: STEPHANIE'S CHILDHOOD

The pain of shame that comes from broken bridges is so great and so threatening to our very survival that we learn to avoid it at all costs. We learn to please, pacify, and lie about our feelings in order to maintain the illusion of connection to other people. I say illusion, because the child who was shamed sufficiently to develop a shame-based identity, a personality organized around self-protection rather than shared mutuality, can no longer form real interpersonal bridges. As children, we learn that the only way to protect against the breaking of bridges is to stop making the bridges. The loneliness and isolation we had hoped to protect ourselves from becomes our constant companion. We end up sealing in the pain we had hoped to seal out. Let's turn to Stephanie's story to understand how this happens.

A strikingly beautiful advertising executive in her early thirties, Stephanie came to see me for help with a serious case of hypochondriasis complicated by a very real problem with asthma. We joked that she was a member of the disease-of-the-month club, but her constant fears that she had cancer, AIDS, or some other life-threatening illness were no laughing matter, nor were the asthma attacks that had plagued her since childhood.

An only child whose mother died suddenly in an accident, the five-year-old Stephanie was left feeling bereft and frightened. Her wealthy, workaholic father, himself the child of shame-based parents, didn't know how to comfort his daughter or himself after his wife died. He took refuge in his work and left Stephanie's care to a nanny. Stephanie spent many lonely nights, waiting with her nanny until eight or nine o'clock, when Daddy came home from the office to spend a few minutes with her. Her father constantly promised he would come home earlier, but usually reneged. Only Stephanie's asthma attacks brought him home from the office early.

After her mother's death, Stephanie's asthma became progressively more severe. While I don't believe that childhood stress and shame create illness, I do believe that they bring out or worsen illness when there is a predilection to it. In these cases, the illness may become an important way for the child to feel close to a parent and receive much-needed care. Illness can become a major source of bonding and bridge-building for a child with an insecure parent, because it provides a safe, predictable structure for parent-child interaction.

As adults, children whose illness served the crucial function of ensuring care and a circumscribed type of closeness often experience worsening of the illness at times when they are stressed, out of control, and in need of emotional support. Their nervous system is conditioned to produce the illness in response to stress because it, in turn, elicits the much-needed caring. In *Minding the Body, Mending the Mind*, we discussed this as a "secondary gain" from illness. The bodymind, in its wisdom, will not let go of an illness whose existence ensures it of the caring so vital to survival. Because of this, finding healthy ways to get emotional needs met is an important part of physical healing for people who have a history like Stephanie's.

All shamed children suffer from emotional abandonment and must find ways to get their needs for bonding met. The death of Stephanie's mother was a traumatic form of abandonment for a five-year-old. Divorce is traumatic as well, particularly when the child is ignored by the parent who leaves, or becomes central to a power struggle. Children often hold themselves responsible for parental illness, divorce, or death, and Stephanie wondered what terrible thing she had done to make her mother leave. Since her father was emotionally unavailable to her, Stephanie had little opportunity to discuss her feelings, which, as we'll see later, is critical to overcoming experiences of trauma and loss. A frightened child who thought of herself as worthless, Stephanie's developing personality organized itself around protecting her from further abandonment. It did this by creating a whole cast of characters, or false selves, designed to gain love and win approval by being as perfect as possible and pleasing in all ways.

Stephanie did whatever was asked of her. She was an excellent student, a good cook, a great protector of her busy father, and prom queen in high school. But as beautiful and talented as Stephanie was as an adult, she attracted only a certain type of man—she called them wolves. "Wolves don't care about you," she told me, "they only want to get what they can out of you—sex, money, or prestige. They're users." The Self in Stephanie was not available to engage the Self in other people and form authentic interpersonal bridges. Instead, her false selves—the multifaceted, inauthentic personality that had been born out of self-protection—sought "counterfeit bridges" by engaging the false self of another person. In dating situations, Stephanie had developed an unconscious radar that allowed the false self she called "femme fatale" to identify and engage wolf personas in her dates. It's not that Stephanie wanted to do this. It happened in spite of her best efforts to the contrary.

Here's how that radar developed. At twelve or thirteen, when Jewish boys and girls of Stephanie's era danced together at Bar Mitzvahs, she had noted that the girls who danced closest were most popular. While Stephanie soon *acted* the role of femme fatale, she developed little capacity for emotional intimacy and had no idea how to handle the flood of sexual feelings that were beginning to arise in her and her young suitors. So she did what she had always done to survive. She tried to please the boys. She became sexually precocious and soon developed a bad reputation. Stephanie's behavior recreated the very feelings of worthlessness she had tried to fend off. In the process, her authentic sexuality was repressed because it had become a source of inner shame.

Reserved and shy despite her impressive array of sophisticated, intellectual, and femme fatale false selves, Stephanie began coming out of her shell a little bit with her first college boyfriend, a sophomore named Steve. She liked him and started to let her defenses down. The Natural

Child in her began to peek through in spontaneous conversation and fun, something that the serious and somewhat rigid Stephanie had already forgotten by the age of eighteen. On their fourth date, they were in Steve's room, kissing and bantering good-humoredly with one another.

I can still remember the happy, dreamy look on her face as she recalled the beginning of the evening that turned into a nightmare. Stephanie liked Steve and thought he cared for her. Even her repressed sexual feelings were beginning to stir. The real Stephanie was coming back to life. Later that evening, when Steve guided her hand to explore his body, she acted authentically with a male for perhaps the very first time. She pulled her hand away, not yet ready for that level of sexual exploration with him. Steve reared back angrily, "Hey, c'mon, Stephanie. I heard you were an easy make in high school. I expected at least a hand-job by the fourth date."

Stephanie was crushed. She cried as she told me how she "shrank back like a sea anemone poked by a stick," feeling totally worthless and humiliated. She felt ashamed, although Steve was the one who acted shamefully. When an interpersonal bridge is broken, the frightened child within us feels as if he or she is to blame, regardless of the circumstance. This was a familiar feeling for Stephanie. The little child in her ached with the old feelings of worthlessness and abandonment that had accompanied her through adolescence and young adulthood and that were still begging for comfort when I met her fifteen years later.

The interpersonal bridge between the two teenagers was totally severed. While it might have been possible for Steve to repair that bridge, he made no attempt to do so. As Stephanie told it, he was a "wolf in sheep's clothing." He had fooled her into trusting him in order to use her. She felt hopelessly betrayed and abused. They never talked again and purposely avoided one another when he came to her dorm to date another girl. Steve's callousness created a scar so deep that Stephanie never again opened the bridge of trust to another man. Although she had dated intermittently, the tendency to attract wolves discouraged her. In her early thirties, Stephanie was effectively married to her career. Like her father before her, she found workaholism a socially acceptable wall behind which to hide her frightened child self.

THE MASK: PSYCHOLOGICAL AND SPIRITUAL MODELS OF THE FALSE SELF

Stephanie's false selves were so familiar to her that they seemed to be who she really was. Yet there's something peculiar about a false self like

Stephanie's femme fatale persona. It's like the image on film of Mae West coming up to a man in a bar and whispering, "Hey there, big boy, come up and see me some time." Stephanie replayed her film clip again and again, and it was always the same. It lacked the nuances of real life. It didn't respond to subtleties in new situations. A false self may look good from a distance, but, on closer inspection, it is rigid and immobile, like a mask. It lacks authenticity and spontaneity. *A mask is a form of compulsive behavior that was adopted in childhood as a way to protect us from the pain of broken bridges*. Although it is maladaptive in adult life, and usually creates new pain, we cannot stop donning it.

My good friend and colleague Robin Casarjian is a therapist and writer who specializes in forgiveness work. She has given the syndrome of renewing our childhood pain by replaying these old roles an impressive clinical name: SSDD—*same stuff, different day*. When our masks continually engage the masks of other people, we are like empty suits of armor jousting. Our behavior is not conscious, but a result of old conditioning. We do not engage each other's true Self and share in the wisdom, joy, peace, and creativity of authentic interpersonal bridges. We can no longer be intimate with another person. Instead we are like shadow boxers or automatons, going through the same motions over and over. We are asleep to who we really are and convinced that we are the familiar roles. This is the case of mistaken identity that forms around shame and gives rise to the behaviors we have characterized as unhealthy guilt.

The concepts of the false self, or mask, that leads to soul sickness, and the true Self whose wisdom enlivens the soul are ancient spiritual concerns. They are central to Eastern philosophies that date back thousands of years. Jesus likewise condemns hypocrisy, a word that derives from a Greek word meaning *one who plays a part*. Since the New Testament was originally written in Greek, we can appreciate the psychological soundness of his words. We will fully discuss the mask and Self as philosophical and spiritual concepts in Chapter Five, when we turn our attention to the timeless question "Who am I?"

While the false self and the true Self were first discussed in philosophical and spiritual circles, they are no less a concern of modern psychological theory. Both mainstream psychoanalytic and eclectic schools of thought view the mask as a defense against vulnerability whose discovery and deposal are critical to the development of personal freedom. Although an extensive review of these theories is beyond our scope, I would like to draw your attention to several theorists whose work has been particularly influential. References can be found in the reading list in Chapter Ten.

Alice Miller, an analyst who has written several compelling books about broken bridges in childhood, including *The Drama of the Gifted Child,* which was originally published under the title *Prisoners of Childhood,* and *For Your Own Good,* traces the history of the mask in psychoanalytic theory:

> Accommodation to parental needs often (but not always) leads to the "as-if personality" (Winnicott has described it as the "false self"). This person develops in such a way that he reveals only what is expected of him, and fuses so completely with what he reveals that—until he comes to analysis—one could scarcely have guessed how much more there is to him, behind this "masked view of himself" (Habermas, 1970). He cannot develop and differentiate his "True self," because he is unable to live it.
>
> —*The Drama of the Gifted Child* [p. 12]

She goes on to discuss the healthy personality as follows:

> I understand a healthy self-feeling to mean the unquestioned certainty that the feelings and wishes one experiences are a part of oneself. . . . This automatic, natural contact with his own emotions and wishes gives an individual strength and self-esteem. He may live out his feelings, be sad, despairing, or in need of help, without fear of making the introjected mother insecure. He can allow himself to be afraid when he is threatened, or angry when his wishes are not fulfilled. He knows not only what he does not want but also what he wants and is able to express this, irrespective of whether he will be loved or hated for it.
>
> —*The Drama of the Gifted Child* [p. 33]

In other words, a healthy person is free to be himself and experience his feelings without worrying about pleasing or displeasing someone else. He can literally be true to his own Self. He can be happy or sad, angry or complacent as he sees fit, rather than pasting on a mask that leaves him feeling anxious, empty, depressed, and out of touch with the true, authentic feelings and impulses that lie beneath. These hidden impulses, the parts of ourselves that we stuff behind the mask, are what Carl Jung called the *shadow* (which we'll soon discuss in this chapter). Virginia Satir, the founding "mother" of family therapy, compared these authentic repressed feelings to a hungry pack of dogs scratching at the cellar door. This is the energy that the mask is restraining and that sometimes breaks through, leaving us with the peculiar feeling that a stranger has moved into our skin. "Why did I do or say or feel that?" we wonder. "Where did that uncharacteristic burst of anger come from?"

The sudden emergence of unfamiliar selves, the shifts in energy, bodily posture, physiology, and moods that we all experience each day intrigued the eclectic psychiatrist Eric Berne in the 1950s. He developed a thoughtful, sensible, and ultimately practical psychological theory and treatment called Transactional Analysis. It is based on the observation that each person moves in and out of different ego states (systems of feelings and accompanying physical reactions and behavior patterns) in his communications, or transactions, with other people and himself. These ego states correspond to parent, child, and adult roles. They can be observed, analyzed, and rendered less compulsive in a way that frees the capability inherent in the wise and creative Natural Child, which Berne endearingly referred to as the "Little Professor."

Berne's recognition that "everyone carries his parents around inside of him" and "everyone carries a little boy or girl around inside of him" are critical for healing our masks and moving beyond the stylized roles we play. Berne called our masklike interactions "rackets" or "scripts" or "games." Stephanie, for example, lived a victim script. The EST training, now called the Forum, developed by Werner Erhardt, is also based on identifying people's lifescripts, or acts, so we can consciously choose to sidestep them.

While all these therapies are psychologically astute and helpful in identifying our masks and analyzing how we came to wear them, they are still only partial approaches to the problem. In my opinion, two things are lacking. First, they identify the problem and create insight into behaviors, but they do not generally touch us where we hurt. Stephanie's adult may understand the origins of her problems with great perspicacity, but when, at age 33, she encounters a situation that reminds her of one she experienced at eight, it's the eight-year-old who needs emotional comfort. No amount of talking to the thirty-three-year-old intellect will make Stephanie feel any better at that moment. No therapy is complete until we learn to comfort ourselves and rebond with the frightened child that is still alive in us as adults. Attempts to do this have arisen primarily out of the Adult Children of Alcoholics movement and are now slowly making their way into the psychological mainstream.

The second lack in most therapies is that they stop at the level of the single bodymind without addressing our connectedness to a larger universal whole. Soul and Spirit are simply left out. In fact, they are kept consciously separate as "religious" concerns that have nothing to do with psychotherapy. This way of thinking was popularized by Sigmund Freud and resulted in the early split between Freud and his spiritual-minded student, Carl Jung. In his essay "The Stages of Life," Jung wrote, "It happens sometimes that I must say to an older patient: 'Your picture of God or your idea of immortality is atrophied, consequently your psychic metabolism is out of gear.' " Without correcting this psychic metabolism, Jung knew, his patients often could not heal.

If we don't go beyond the *intrapersonal* realm of our relation to our own Self and the *interpersonal* realm of our relationships with others, we ignore the basic connection of all human beings with a larger Source of being. This is called the *transpersonal* realm. A thoughtful and elegant form of transpersonal psychotherapy was conceptualized in the early 1900s by Italian psychiatrist Roberto Assagioli, who was a contemporary and colleague of Freud and Jung. It is called psychosynthesis.

Psychosynthesis is based on identifying the largely unconscious and reflexive false selves (what Assagioli calls subpersonalities) and reintegrating them back into a conscious whole where they serve the Self and enrich the wisdom that is stored in our soul. In assuming and discussing the existence of the soul and its relationship to the Spirit, psychosynthesis goes beyond psychology's concept of the personal self. Assagioli based his system on the philosophical view that each person *has* a superficial and somewhat changeable personality necessary for functioning in this world, but *is* an enduring and immortal soul whose growing wisdom is added to by the experiences of a lifetime. These views are part of what scientist and philosopher Aldous Huxley called the *perennial philosophy*, that core set of beliefs that are reiterated in the wisdom traditions of all cultures and represent a kind of collective world wisdom unchanging through the ages.

In order to break through the collection of false selves, we need to reown the vitality of the Natural Child. The question is, where did all that exuberance go? What happened to the boundless energy of childhood? The usual explanation that energy dissipates as the body ages is more a rationalization than a biological fact. We have all experienced the tremendous energy that accompanies a creative rush when we are planning a vacation, a garden, a painting, a poem, or any creative or exciting project that gets us "in gear." We have all experienced the exhaustion of giving up.

Physical energy varies with mental state. There is usually more energy in reserve than we are using. So where is it? Carl Jung told us to look for it in all the disowned parts of ourselves that we offered to our parents but they didn't want. We took these gifts and hid them away in what Jung called the *shadow*. Reowning the shadow gives us the energy we need to undertake the journey of rediscovering the Self and our eternal natures both as part of the Spirit and as personalities experiencing the joys and sorrows of a lifetime. Only then can we fully realize the wisdom and creativity that are expressions of the unique potential of our own soul. Only then are we really capable of loving and being loved.

THE SHADOW: THE LONG BAG WE DRAG BEHIND US

Robert Bly, an American poet, compares the shadow to a long bag we drag behind us. In it are all the parts of us that our parents didn't like, our teachers considered naughty, our clergy branded unholy, and so forth. In it is every natural impulse and emotion that has ever been shamed.

The shadow contains the vital energy of the Natural Child that may have been shamed in rebelliousness, sexuality, spontaneity, excitement, and even the need to rest, daydream, and create, which may have been criticized as laziness. Perhaps the shadow will come alive for you in a story about a long bag of my own, one that I literally dragged down the road for most of one dark, moonless night when attempting to run away from camp and find my way back home at a tender, young age. Although they made me unpack the bag after my capture, I kept a ghostly double of it with me for most of my life. In it, I stuffed all the things that were branded bad about my abortive flight to freedom, and hence myself. Here's what happened.

I was only seven years old when I was sent to a supposedly exclusive overnight camp for eight weeks, away from home for the first time. I was a year younger than the other girls in my bunk and fair game for their nasty little pranks. My tennis balls were thrown into the woods, they short-sheeted my bed, and I was forced to play patient in their secret games of doctor. The counselor in charge was what my sons call a nerd. She just told me to shut up and mind my own business when I complained about the pranks and games. So, one dark, moonless night, I stuffed all my belongings into a duffel bag and ran away, dragging the heavy green sack behind me.

I was caught just after dawn, trying to call home from a phone booth in a little country store by the side of the long, dusty road that led out to the highway. Hauled back to the camp grounds, I was stood up on a lunch table where the camp director made a spectacle of me—a public humiliation. Next I was locked up alone in the bunk house all day every day except for meals—for the remaining four weeks of the summer! I played a lot of jacks. Letters to my parents were censored "for my protection," for I was told that if my family ever found out what I'd done I'd be in real trouble. At the age of seven, I thought that I'd ruined my life and was beyond redemption. It never occurred to me that I'd stumbled into a surrealistic concentration camp where the adults were stark raving mad! I can only imagine how physically or sexually abused children must feel, and wonder how they could possibly endure the intensity of the shame.

It took many years for me to find out what had been permanently stuffed into the long bag of my shadow that summer long ago. My camp experience taught me it was not only bad, but absolutely dangerous to stand up to authority. Courage was an offense punishable by emotional death and literal imprisonment. Courage went into my bag. That summer I also learned that telling the truth was useless and perceived as "bad" when the bunkmate who was your worst tormentor was the camp director's niece. A piece of my integrity went into the bag. That summer I learned that being your own person was the worst mistake you could ever make. My selfhood went into the bag. I have spent the rest of my life trying to pull myself back out of the bag.

Everyone's personal bag contains a different mixture of forbidden fruits, although we share a communal shadow with our peers. In the 1960s, for example, my friends and I put our bras, girdles, and high-heeled shoes into the bag. Shaved legs, permanent waves, and love of money went in next as we became full members of the hippie generation. Many of us still can't help apologizing to one another for new cars and nice clothes if we have them! After all, in the sixties such items were shameful symbols of the materialism that was supposed to stay in the bag.

Throughout our childhood and early adult years we continue to fill the bag. After it is full, and we are heavily weighed down, the burden starts to become noticeable. Then we begin to empty the bag. In doing so, we reown our lost power and lighten our load. *But if we do not reown that power, it will begin to work against us, often with serious consequences.* As Robert Bly puts it:

> We spend our life until we're twenty deciding what parts of ourself to put into the bag, and we spend the rest of our lives trying to get

> them out again. Sometimes retrieving them feels impossible, as if the bag were sealed. Suppose the bag remains sealed—what happens then? A great nineteenth-century story has an idea about that. One night Robert Louis Stevenson woke up and told his wife a bit of a dream he'd just had. She urged him to write it down; he did, and it became "Dr. Jekyll and Mr. Hyde." The nice side of our personality becomes, in our idealistic culture, nicer and nicer. The Western man may be a liberal doctor, for example, always thinking about the good of others. Morally and ethically he is wonderful. But the substance in the bag takes on a life of its own; it can't be ignored. The story says that the substance locked in the bag appears one day *somewhere else* in the city. The substance in the bag feels angry . . . when we put a part of ourselves in the bag it regresses. It de-volves toward barbarism.
>
> —*A Little Book on the Human Shadow* [pp. 18–19]

So, while we're sporting the masks of niceness and conformity, our courage, impulsiveness, freedom, sexuality, anger, and so forth are building up a head of steam, getting wilder and wilder inside us. They become dangerous because they live in darkness, informing our behaviors without our consciously knowing they are there. They can express themselves quite suddenly and explosively in "accidents," impulsive behavior, illnesses or lapses of judgment involving errors that are out of character for us. They express themselves chronically in Casarjian's SSDD syndrome: same stuff, different day. In other words, an unexplored shadow leaves us stuck without understanding why, assaulted by strange impulses, and powerless to change.

You may be wondering, then, how on earth we can get those parts of ourselves back out of the bag before they explode. If we are unconscious of the contents of the bag, how can we see what's in there? The unconscious, in its wisdom, leaves us clues about its contents in the psychological defense mechanism called *projection*. If little Sally is burning up with envy over Susie's new doll, but envy has already been stuck in the bag, Sally cannot admit or even experience envy as her own feeling. But it *is* safe to see envy in someone else. So Sally goes up to Jane and comments on *her* jealousy, explaining that not everybody can have a new doll like Susie. Sally has taken her own disowned feeling and projected it outside of herself by seeing it in Jane.

In projection, we see the hidden, "shameful" parts of ourselves in someone else. I was once at a business meeting with a colleague who, while a very anxious person (although these feelings were split off into his shadow), always tried to maintain an air of complete control and composure (his mask). I found the meeting pretty dull and nearly nodded off, but it obviously awakened some anxiety in Sam, since he commented on how anxious *I'd* been the whole time! There's an old saying about the shadow: *What we can tolerate the least in here is what we see the most out there*.

Projection is the basis of self-righteousness and scapegoating. The latter term involves punishing other people for what we have mistakenly labeled as evil in ourselves. In her chilling book *For Your Own Good: Hidden Cruelty in Child-Rearing and the Roots of Violence*, Alice Miller argues that the German people—traditionally raised to strictly repress feelings—were psychologically susceptible to Hitler's scapegoating of the Jews. The Jews were a repository for the projection of a whole nation's shadow. The sad irony is that violence against others is almost always an externalization of violence against ourselves. This is the danger of the unexplored shadow. In Part Three of this book, we will explore ways to reown the contents of the shadow when we consider the dynamics of forgiveness and healing through conscious relationships.

A SUMMARY OF THE INNER CHILD'S DRAMA

> The drama is this. We came as infants "trailing clouds of glory," arriving from the farthest reaches of the universe, bringing with us appetites well preserved from our mammal inheritance, spontaneities wonderfully preserved from our 150,000 years of tree life, angers well preserved from our 5,000 years of tribal life—in short with our 360 degree radiance—and we offered this gift to our parents. They didn't want it. They wanted a nice girl or a nice boy. That's the first act of the drama.
>
> —Robert Bly, *A Little Book on the Human Shadow* [p. 24]

In the acts that follow, we put on the mask of the false self that we think our parents want, store our leftover glory in the bag, and then become exhausted and disheartened because we are empty of ourselves. From time to time, grace (the messenger of the Spirit) knocks on the door with a telegram that says something is wrong. Perhaps our headaches get worse, our marriage breaks up, or we start to drink or take drugs. Since we have free will, we can heed these messages or ignore them. If we ignore them, we get progressively more miserable and desperate. If we heed them and become aware of our shame-based false self and the unhealthy guilt it creates, we enter the healing phase.

William James used a medical metaphor to describe the two ways that people heal back into the Self and discover their connection to the Spirit. In some people, healing is a slow process of *lysis*, a gradual dissolution of the false identity. For others, healing takes the form of *crisis*. In crisis, we find ourselves in a face-to-face confrontation with the inner demons that have been growing strong and cunning in the bag. The more controlling we are, the harder it is to let go so as to see our shadow gradually, and the likelihood increases that we will heal by crisis. In crisis, we quickly learn that we cannot win alone. We need the help of friends and the grace of God. In our healing, we learn to ask for help.

A Review of Who We Are, Who We Thought We Were, and Why We Thought We Were Somebody That We Aren't!

1. The universal consciousness, or lifeforce, is present within each human being as the Self.

2. The Natural Child, or soul at birth, is filled with the creativity, wisdom, love, joy, enthusiasm, and contentment that radiate from the Self. We call this state of being happiness and authenticity. Happiness is the substance of our soul and a reflection of the greater Spirit from which our individual consciousness springs. Happiness is inborn. It cannot be learned, but it *can* be forgotten. Authenticity is an attitude of awareness in which we are willing to experience our thoughts and feelings as they are.

3. The interpersonal bridge of love is a link between the Self and souls of two human beings. Self-to-Self bridges create a state of mutuality in which two people mirror each other's states of mind and together experience a deeper emotion, wisdom, creativity, and joy than either usually experiences alone. *This state of soul-union, in which we reconnect with Spirit through sharing with another human being, is love.*

4. If the Self of a parent, because of past hurts, is generally unavailable to connect with a child's Self, a "pseudo" or "counterfeit" connection will be made instead through one of the parent's false selves. Because the masks of the false self are rigid, they preclude mutuality of experience, which consists of a moment-to-moment flow of emotion and the mirroring of two people's inner states. For example, a father playing tennis

with his twelve-year-old son may be wearing a "teacher" mask. All will go well unless the child begins to win, refuses to play, or in any way violates the teacher mask's rigid rules. The father may then shame his son and break the bridge. The "love" in the interaction was conditional on the child conforming to his father's preconceptions.

5. Conditional love breeds shame. Shame is an adaptive, submissive state that favors survival but creates fear and helplessness. When the interpersonal bridge is severed through shame, the child feels as if he is in mortal danger. He is humiliated and enraged but is powerless to express his rage.

6. Shame is the master emotion because it has the power to determine which other emotions we can feel. Gershen Kaufman traces this process to the *affect-shame bind*. An affect is a primary emotional state such as interest, enjoyment, surprise, anger, distress, shame, or disgust. *Whenever a child's expression of an affect is shamed, that affect is quickly stuffed into the bag.* For example, little Bobby screams for Mommy one night because the shirt draped over the back of his chair looks like a terrible monster. Mommy comes and belittles Bobby for being a silly crybaby. Bobby sticks fear in the bag, but not only fear of shirt-monsters. All kinds of unrelated fears go into his shadow as well, because the original fear-shame bind was so powerful. Pretty soon Bobby forgets how to feel fear, or he begins to call it something else—maybe anger or even boredom. Through affect-shame binds, our emotional life gets numb, confused, or both.

7. We develop masks in response to conditional love and the shame that it creates. There are an endless variety of masks worn to purchase affection or protection, or to just numb our pain. Developed in childhood, masks are survival strategies that become the unconscious directors of our thoughts, emotions, and behaviors. Some common masks for our insecurities are people-pleasing, being a victim, seductiveness, control-oriented behaviors, manipulation, perfectionism, religious zealotry, superachieving, raging, rescuing, patronizing, being self-righteous, and becoming an addict. These masks give rise to the shame-based thoughts, emotions, and behaviors that we call unhealthy guilt.

8. The more we have been shamed, the longer our shadow and the more rigid our masks. Since our masks cover over the Self and obscure the knowledge in our soul, our capacity for joy, peace, wisdom, creativity, and happiness gets submerged, and we lose touch with our real nature.

We become one-dimensional caricatures who lack the normal depth of human feeling. We may think we can feel emotions, but more likely we are ruled by the rage and fear of our inner child. Positive emotions are rarely experienced, and we cannot be fully present in life. We have lost much of our capacity for self-awareness and suffer from perilously low self-esteem.

9. We are all somewhere along the continuum between identifying with our false self and realizing our eternal Self. Our place along the continuum is not a value judgment about how good or smart or clever or spiritual we are. It is just where we are. Knowing where we are is the first step to healing.

THE INNER CHILD'S GUIDANCE

The drama of the child is both psychological and spiritual. The drama involves the personality as we know it psychologically and its reflection in mask and shadow. The drama also involves the soul, which is developing wisdom and a richness of experience even as we form our false selves. The problem we have is not in becoming wise, but in accessing that wisdom. Since the false self forms a veil or sheath around the soul (what psychologists call defenses), we only vaguely see what is beneath. Nonetheless, the soul's wisdom continues to guide us in the same way that the sun still lights our way when it's behind the clouds.

I was ten years old when I had a particularly trying dark night of the soul. Within a short period of time, we had moved and the nanny who, like a mother, had raised me left to marry. I felt abandoned and frightened of being rejected by a new peer group. I felt as if the rug had been pulled out from under me, and I lost my bearings. I went into a deep depression that lasted for the better part of a year. For several weeks, I was too afraid to attend school. I was plagued by nightmares for months.

In the worst part of my terror I wrote a poem, or rather my Natural Child did. Even in our darkest hours we are never alone. Grace brings about breaks in the clouds where the Self can shine through and illumine the soul's wisdom. If we look for and value the little messages that peek through the clouds, we will have gifts to sustain us through the child's inner journey. Here is the gift that my Natural Child gave to me in the midst of that great darkness. It has been an inspiration and a comfort to me in hard times for nearly thirty-five years. Perhaps it may lighten your way a little as well.

The Light

Somewhere in the darkest night
There always shines
A small, bright Light.
This light up in the heavens shines
To help our God watch over us.
When a small child is born
The Light his soul does adorn.
But when our only human eyes
Look up in the lightless skies
We always know
Even though we can't quite see
That a little Light
Burns far into the night
To help our God watch over us.

SUGGESTIONS FOR THE READER

1. Can you recognize any of your false selves? Do you know when they formed? Author Megan LeBoutillier recalls the birth of her "Little Miss Perfect." It happened one day when she fell into the toilet and spoiled her party dress at age four. Little Miss Perfect was born out of her shame and the determination to avoid such a painful situation ever again.

2. When you gave birth to a false self, you stuffed some part of you into your shadow. What emotions or attitudes are composting in that long, heavy bag? One way to discover what is in there is to pay attention to your projections. What is it that bothers you the most about other people? What characteristics are common to several people whom you dislike?

CHAPTER FOUR

Healing the Inner Child

Inside me there is a seven-year-old who is still hurting from her humiliation at summer camp. Her anguish is reawakened every time I find myself in the presence of an authority figure who acts in a controlling manner. At those moments, my intellect is prone to desert me, and I am liable to break down and cry with the same desolation and helplessness I felt when I was seven.

Were you ever surprised by feeling overwhelmed with hurt and anger when someone forgot to call you or acted insensitively toward you? Were you ever panicked for no good reason? Did you ever wake up depressed and not know why? Not only do childhood's wounds cause us to experience emotions out of context or out of proportion to a current situation, they may also prevent us from experiencing our emotions at all.

Emotions that we cannot allow into consciousness often express themselves somatically, through our body. Consider the case of Barry, a lawyer in his late twenties who came to me for help with severe lower-back pain. At our first meeting, Barry shared something with me that really perplexed him. The youngest and favorite of three children, he described his relationship to his mother as "exceptionally close." Yet when his mother died suddenly of a heart attack, Barry felt nothing at all. He could not grieve.

Six months after her death, the "little twinges" that Barry had felt in his back for years developed into serious, disabling pain. That's when Barry came for help. His physical pain did not begin to lessen until he faced the emotional pain of his childhood. Barry was not "close" to his mother in the sense of authentic bridges; he was engulfed by her smothering, conditional love. Only when he began to mourn for his lost self and to feel the hidden rage that he had carried in his shadow for years could he begin to forgive his mother and to grieve for her. Only then did his back pain go away.

We cannot begin to heal the wounded inner child and recover from our shame and unhealthy guilt until, like Barry, we understand what the child is feeling. When emotional energy is blocked and is prevented from flowing in its natural channels, it gets stored in our body as tension and pain. When emotional energy is bound up, we are also robbed of a crucial information and emergency-mobilization network.

> Our emotions are part of our basic power. They serve two major functions in our psychic life. They monitor our basic needs, telling us of a need, a loss or a satiation. Without our emotional energy, we would not be aware of our most fundamental needs. Emotions also give us the fuel or energy to act. I like to hyphenate the word E-motion. An E-motion is energy in motion. This energy moves us to get what we need. When our basic needs are being violated, our anger moves us to fight or run.
>
> —John Bradshaw, *Healing the Shame That Binds You* [p. 52]

LETTING BOUND EMOTIONS OUT OF THE BAG

A critical part of healing our wounded children and recovering our lost vitality is unloading the emotions that are hidden in our bag. Remember that the contents of the bag have been composting, getting wilder and wilder. Anger stuffed in the bag becomes rage. Fear stuck in the bag becomes panic. Sadness stuck in the bag becomes paralyzing grief or emotional numbness. Keep this in mind and expect that you will relive very powerful emotions as you begin your healing. This is not craziness, it is the beginning of sanity. But it is painful. There is no way to avoid facing the pain that is still locked inside.

Because shadow emotions are strong, we need the help of supportive others who can listen to us with compassion and allow us to express what we feel. Good listeners can hear empathetically without belittling, dictating what we should or shouldn't feel, cutting us short by dispensing advice, or trying to comfort us instead of hearing us out. Good listeners can be family members, friends, therapists, or members of different types of support or therapy groups. Twelve-step programs like Overeaters Anonymous, Alcoholics Anonymous, Alanon, Adult Children of Alcoholics, and the growing number of spin-offs are another good place for some of us to get appropriate support.

In the remainder of this chapter and in some of the chapters to come, there are experiential exercises meant to increase your awareness of shadow material, comfort the inner child, or lead to new insight. I think of these as Inner Wisdom Exercises, because they free your Natural Child and help you tap the wisdom that the Self embodies. While many readers will find these exercises interesting and enlightening, some of the exercises will naturally reconnect you to old pain. If you were an abused child or had a particularly traumatic childhood, you may not want to stir up that pain unless you are in therapy. There are other reasons why you may not want to encounter old pain at this time in your life. All the exercises are optional in the sense that you don't need to do them to understand the general point I am making or to use the remainder of the book to full advantage. Doing or not doing the exercises is your own personal choice.

INNER WISDOM EXERCISES FOR HEALING THE INNER CHILD

The most important thing about any exercise you do, here or elsewhere, is to let go of any expectations you might have about what is supposed to happen. You can never know in advance.

Expectations create limitations and unhealthy guilt when you don't get what you want or you get what you don't want! Any kind of inner wisdom exercise may lead to amazing insights, great relief, anxiety, delight, upset, sadness, peace, rage, wisdom, boredom, or nothing at all. In short, our experiences reflect the entire range of human emotion. This is exactly the point of such exercises. They are not meant to make you nicer or more "positive," or to reinforce any expected quality. They are meant to let you feel what you are feeling and to be who you are. Without any attachment to the outcome, you can feel good about whatever happens or doesn't happen. The ability to let yourself have experiences without their conforming to expectation is itself evidence of healing.

EXERCISE: RESTORING BRIDGES TO THE INNER CHILD

Stop for a moment. Take a few letting-go breaths—nice big sighs of relief—and close your eyes. Now think back to the last time you were really upset beyond what the situation called for or were confused about what you were feeling. *When you have a situation clearly in mind, you are ready to do an exercise to contact your inner child.* You may discover a shamed emotion from your past and restore the broken interpersonal bridge by listening to, accepting, and comforting your inner child. Keep this incident in mind as you read about the purpose of the exercise and the instructions for doing it.

The purpose of the following exercise is to allow the old emotions that are adding to your current difficulty to come to consciousness. Those emotions got stuffed in your bag during childhood when you were shamed for having them. The inner child is still hurting from those unresolved incidents. During the exercise, you can travel back in time, guided by the hidden emotional energy, to a scene from your childhood when shaming or other important events occurred. Your own inner wisdom will select an appropriate memory from the vast stores of your unconscious. You can then give your child the unconditional love it needs to feel good, literally "correcting" the old memory. In this way, some of the emotional energy bound by shame is freed.

You can read these instructions and then do the exercise yourself, or have someone read the instructions to you, or tape them and play them back to yourself using the pronoun him or her as appropriate. The whole exercise takes three to five minutes.

Take a few letting-go breaths and close your eyes. Your breath is the link between past and present, conscious and unconscious, the adult and the child. . . . In your mind's eye see the number three. . . . As you exhale, let the three dissolve and become a two. . . . As you exhale, let the two dissolve and become a one. . . . As you exhale, let the one dissolve and become a zero. Let the zero elongate into an oval mirror, and in it you will see yourself in a scene from your childhood. What is happening? Ask your childself what he is experiencing and how he feels. Listen with great respect and love. . . . When the child is finished, tell him what he needs to hear. . . . Take a minute to comfort him. You may want to pick the child up, hug him, or stroke his hair. Do what is needed to restore the child's sense of self, to repair the bridge that was broken. Reassure the child and give him love. Let him know that you will be back to talk again, and that he can count on you for love and understanding, no matter what. When you are ready, release the child into the mirror and let the mirror collapse back into a circle. Let the circle become a one, the one become a two and the two become a three. Open your eyes and come back to the room.

What happened? If you found yourself as a child, comforted yourself, and restored the bridge, you probably felt relief. Maybe you even felt love. Perhaps you felt some pain or had an insight. Did you find out what emotion was bound? If nothing at all happened, that's fine, too. Your unconscious may provide you with insight later, in a dream, as a sudden flash, or in the attraction to a certain book. If you did learn something about yourself or experience something of interest, even though it may not have made sense, take a minute and make a few notes about it in your journal or any little notebook.

I originally learned the technique of using the mirror countdown to access unconscious wisdom from Dr. Harriett Mann, a therapist in Cambridge, Massachusetts. You can ask the "magic mirror" about anything at all. It serves as a conduit to both personal and transpersonal stores of wisdom and memory. I have taught this exercise to thousands of people at workshops around the country, and I am always amazed at the variety of interesting revelations that people have. Each time you do a magic mirror exercise, you are building a skill. After several tries, you may find that "going inside" to find your child or become receptive to other information becomes second nature. You may find that you revisit the same scene or the same age several times or enter a different scene each time. The child you find may be an infant or even a young adult. Whenever you contact the entity psychiatrist Dr. Hugh Missildine, a pioneer in inner child work, has called an *inner child of the past*, you have the opportunity to finish old business by comforting the child's pain and consciously absorbing whatever learning the situation had to offer. In this way, you can help set yourself free not by erasing the past, but by placing it in a larger context where your own compassion and care form a new frame of reference for the old pattern, thereby transforming it.

EXERCISE: VISITING THE INNER CHILD ON A REGULAR BASIS

You can extend the benefits of contacting, communicating with, and comforting the inner child by doing so regularly. You can repeat the exercise above whenever you need insight into confusing situations or emotional binds, or when old patterns are preventing you from acting freely.

You can also visit with your inner child on a daily basis. Many people find the following practice both a comforting way to start the day and a powerful practice for healing the past. In the morning when you wake up, while you're still underneath the covers, take a few deep breaths or use the magic mirror. Bring to mind a place from your childhood where you remember feeling safe. If you can't remember a safe place from your childhood, imagine one as you would have liked it to be. Greet your child there. Ask what her anticipations are for the day to come. *Listen with respect and caring to whatever she says rather than trying to talk her out of any painful feelings that she may express.* Let the child know that you hear and understand her concerns, then respond verbally, if it's required. You may also want to ask her advice about the upcoming day, tapping the innate wisdom of your Natural Child. Before you leave, spend a moment just hugging and caring for the child. Look into her eyes. Make a bridge of love and trust. Let her know that you'll be back.

Repeat the exercise before you go to sleep at night. Go back inside your imagination to that safe place and review the day with your child, listening to her feelings, comforting her and talking to her. Remember that you can also ask her for advice. Eric Berne called the Natural Child the Little Professor for good reason. The child is a wise adviser whom you can really grow to appreciate.

ILLNESS AND THE INNER CHILD

One of my patients, a woman named Martha, got into bed one afternoon with a bad bellyache—a symptom of the spastic colon she'd had for years. Martha had been doing inner child work for a few weeks and decided to find and comfort the little "Martie"—usually a four-year-old. When Martha went into her imagination, she was surprised to find a baby of ten or eleven months sitting on the floor, all alone and crying inconsolably. She instinctively scooped up the baby, sat down in a rocking chair, and began to nurse her. Resting in this image for several minutes, Martha gradually became aware that, as she was comforting the baby, her gut was relaxing and the pain was going away.

The next time Martha's gut went into spasm, she went right back inside and found the baby. Once again, nursing her for several minutes cured the pain. There was a very young part of Martha—a preverbal part of her—that was frightened about not getting her most basic needs of love and sustenance met. For several months, Martha visited the baby regularly and cared for her with love and affection. Gradually her colon condition disappeared, and one day so did the baby, replaced by the four-year-old with whom Martha had begun her inner child work months before.

Martha was not unusual in discovering that a physical illness was related to the unmet needs of her inner child. While it is important to realize that illness occurs for many different reasons that may or may not be influenced by childhood experience, psychologist James Pennebaker at Southern Methodist University has reviewed a large body of scientific literature indicating that adults who experienced childhood trauma are more likely to develop diseases ranging from high blood pressure and ulcers to cancer than those without such early traumas. This research does not mean that childhood trauma causes illness. It means that trauma is one factor out of many that increase the chance of illness occurring. Without a genetic predisposition or an environmental cause, the most traumatic childhood cannot elevate the risk of disease, other than for those conditions directly related to stress and anxiety, such as muscle-tension headaches, digestive disturbances, and some cardiovascular problems. My own experience is a case in point.

When I returned home from the summer camp I told you about, I steadfastly guarded my secret shame over running away, terrified of being found out and chastised. Then one day the following winter, as my parents discussed sending me back to the camp for a second year, I could stand it no more and let out my terrible secret. My parents couldn't believe it. They had researched several camps and done their best to choose a good one. In their shock and disbelief, they did what many parents do when episodes of abuse are uncovered. They assumed that I was making up at least part of the story and overdramatizing the rest. These things simply don't happen, do they?

While I was relieved not to be punished and to be spared from attending the camp again, I was very sad not to be fully believed. I had lots of bad dreams and soon developed blinding migraine headaches that continued for nearly twenty years, ceasing only when I learned the mind/body skills of meditation and creative imagination described in *Minding the Body, Mending the Mind*. Only in recent years did I discover that an incipient headache could be aborted not only by meditation, but that it could be stopped even faster by going inside and comforting the seven-year-old Joanie who had been abused at that camp.

Fortunately, most of us are spared from the truly humiliating experience of abuse and its attendant shame, but whenever a child is not taken seriously by her parents, whenever her creative efforts or feelings are belittled or discounted, shame occurs as the little shock of nonrecognition and nonacceptance reverberates through the nervous system.

Every human being encounters traumas, losses, and disappointments in life that leave us feeling bad—sad, angry, hurt, vulnerable, betrayed, or frightened. We seek to understand the causes of our suffering and to learn what we can, most naturally by talking to other people about our troubles. Unfortunately, many upsetting situations are hard to discuss. Victims of childhood sexual abuse and physical abuse and children from alcoholic homes are often ashamed of their stories, as I was, and may hold back. Unfortunately, it takes physiological energy as well as mental energy to deny, to inhibit the pain that yearns for comforting. As we've seen, when that bound-up emotional energy interacts with an underlying physical weakness, disease can result. This is what happened in the case of my headaches, Barry's back pain, and Martha's irritable bowel syndrome.

Drs. James Pennebaker and Sandra Beall did a revealing experiment with forty-six college students concerning the relation between unexpressed emotion and illness. They hypothesized that since denial of feelings requires active inhibition and real physiological work, thus generating stress, they should be able to trace health differences in students who disclosed their feelings about traumas compared to those who didn't. They devised an experiment in which students wrote about different experiences during four consecutive evenings. Physiological measures of fight-or-flight, such as blood pressure and heart rate, were made directly after writing, and the students' health was measured for the following six months.

A control group was assigned trivial writing exercises; they were requested, for instance, to write essays about their shoes. Another group wrote about their traumas, but only about the facts—no feelings. The rest of the students wrote about the trauma *and* their feelings. The third group, the emotional disclosers, responded with fight-or-flight and higher blood pressures directly after the writing, and they felt more distressed the next day. But six months later, the emotional disclosers reported fewer symptoms and visited physicians for illness significantly fewer times than students in the other groups. When queried about whether the experiment had any long-lasting effects, the disclosers responded very positively, citing greater insight, less tension, more peace of mind, and an ability to think about things that were previously too painful to accept.

Many spontaneously took up journal writing as a way to extend these benefits.

Contacting the inner child is a very direct way of relieving the pain, processing feelings, and dealing with old traumas. As Pennebaker and Beall showed, writing about our experiences helps, as does talking them through with a good listener. But dealing with feelings bound up in the past is only part of the healing work we need to do. Because we were not allowed certain feelings as children, we cannot recognize them easily now. In addition to correcting old traumas, we must also sharpen our skills in recognizing current emotions. To do this, we must learn how to listen to ourselves with respect.

LEARNING TO LISTEN

Learning to listen to ourselves is a way of learning to love ourselves, just as listening to other people is a powerful form of love. In my workshops, I often have participants do a listening exercise adapted from a psychotherapy teaching exercise that I learned from psychologist Bob Ginn, a family therapist in Cambridge, Massachusetts. The exercise is simplicity itself. Two strangers pair up, and one begins to talk—about anything at all. The other must sit *silently*, listening with great attention and respect but saying nothing. After ten minutes, the two change roles and the talker becomes the listener. When the time is up and the two can talk to each other, it's like witnessing a reunion of old friends! Most people start their ten-minute soliloquy with the weather and end up talking about deep hopes and fears. There's something about the respectful silence and attention of the listener that brings out feelings that need comfort or affirmation.

One of the most common frustrations of the listeners is the injunction they receive against saying empathetic things or giving advice. Most of us think that other people will find us rude if we don't reply and that they won't like us. Yet the experience in the listening exercise is just the opposite. The talker usually reports that he felt deep empathy and didn't really want any advice; in fact, it probably would have interfered with the empathetic bonding that occurred. People often comment that they haven't felt as close to another human being in years. The trust and care that builds up between two strangers in twenty minutes is really remarkable. Respectful listening creates a strong interpersonal bridge.

The experience of respectful listening is also something we can do for ourselves. It has several benefits. First, it increases awareness of emotions. Whenever you are feeling anxious or empty—what we often just call bad or out of sorts—real feelings are just beneath conscious awareness, stuck in the shadow. Second, listening to ourselves is a way of caring for ourselves that increases self-esteem. Third, respectful listening is a way to reparent ourselves and to rebuild bridges that were severed when our true feelings were not accepted as children. Here are four simple steps to improve your self-listening skills:

Step One: Respectful Listening

Stop and zero in on what you are actually feeling. If the emotion is not obvious, ask questions to help direct your attention to its source. For example, if you are feeling restless or bored, ask yourself what the restlessness is all about. What led up to it? What were you thinking? What do you really need right now that you haven't got? Maybe the restlessness will turn out to be anxiety, anger, or some creative urge that needs expression. Keep open to the inquiry. If you can't actually feel an emotion or identify a need, ask yourself, "What could I do right now that would make me feel better?"

Step Two: Accepting Your Feelings

Stay open to any feeling that surfaces. "Ah, anger. How interesting." Don't tell yourself that it's bad or try to make it go away. You don't have to do a thing about how you feel other than accept it. Focus your awareness on the feeling and flow along wherever it takes you. It may take you into the body, where you notice fear or tension. It may take you back to old memories. It may take you back to a rerun of the situation that provoked it. It doesn't matter where it takes you, or even if it reveals its source. Trust that if this insight is to be helpful, it will come as part of the process. If it isn't, it won't.

Step Three: Comforting Yourself

How good it feels to have someone hold you when you're feeling bad. You can do this for yourself by taking a few deep sighs of relief to help let go of mental tension, then directing a flow of loving feelings toward yourself. Close your eyes and imagine yourself as a little child, as we did earlier. Then you can pick up the child and hold it close, stroking its hair, rocking it, crooning to it, or comforting it in the way that feels best to you. With practice, it will get easier and easier to feel love and acceptance for yourself. Sooner or later, you'll be able to access loving feelings directly, without necessarily needing to call them up through the exercise of imagining your inner child.

Step Four: Checking to See If the Process Is Complete

After you have listened to your feelings and accepted yourself, the process may be complete. If your body feels relaxed and you are peaceful, then a natural letting go has occurred. But if you still feel physically or mentally tense, then the process isn't yet complete. Take a few letting-go breaths and go back inside your imagination to find your child. Comfort it and then ask it lovingly what it needs to feel better. You may get a direct answer and you may not. The experience will be different every time, so go into it without expectations.

Although our bridges may have been broken many times, as a child and as an adult, when we practice respectful listening we can rebuild bridges. In listening to our own inner child and our own adult self, we actually take part in a process of reparenting ourselves that will lead to the emotional independence that allows us to be authentically who we are. We will also become better at listening to others with the same patience, love, and respect we have learned to extend to ourselves.

LOVE'S EPILOGUE ON GROWING UP

The process of separating from our parents and becoming ourselves is never easy. The more we have been raised with conditional love, the harder it is, since we really and truly don't know where our parents end and we begin. We don't know what is in our shadow and who we are beneath our mask. Even if we were very fortunate and had love in our childhood that was largely unconditional, it is still hard to leave the nest and go out on our own. This painful period of announcing our fledgling independence is called adolescence. It is often a turbulent time because sorting out our dreams and values from those of our parents requires that we take risks, make mistakes, and establish new sets of boundaries between our parents and ourselves. In adolescence, we take the first steps on a lifelong journey of becoming ourselves and finding our highest potential and greatest happiness.

At fifteen, as I struggled through a particularly stormy and confusing adolescence, my father gave me a copy of *The Prophet* by Kahlil Gibran. Sitting together in the den one rainy Sunday afternoon, he read to me the Prophet's teaching about children and parents. His soft and gentle eyes filled with tears as we shared the pain of separation that is an inevitable part of growing up, and as we celebrated the joy of sharing life together. He died when I was thirty, and I have missed the opportunities to share some of my postadolescent growing up with him and to share in his growing old. He was a wonderful man. This is what he read to me on that bittersweet afternoon so long ago.

On Children

And a woman who held a babe against
her bosom said, Speak to us of Children.
And he said:
Your children are not your children.
They are the sons and daughters of Life's
longing for itself.
They come through you but not from
you,
And though they are with you yet they
belong not to you.

You may give them your love but not
your thoughts,
For they have their own thoughts.
You may house their bodies but not
their souls,
For their souls dwell in the house of
tomorrow, which you cannot visit, not even
in your dreams.
You may strive to be like them, but seek
not to make them like you.
For life goes not backward nor tarries
with yesterday.

You are the bows from which your
children as living arrows are sent forth.
The archer sees the mark upon the path
of the infinite, and He bends you with His
might that His arrows may go swift and far.
Let your bending in the archer's hand
be for gladness;
For even as He loves the arrow that flies,
so he loves also the bow that is stable.

Remember this, both as you may parent other people, and as you must inevitably learn to parent yourself.

SUGGESTIONS FOR THE READER

1. If you feel comfortable doing them, try the inner child exercises. Write down a few notes about your experiences in your journal or a little notebook.

2. Practice respectful listening to feelings, both your own and those of other people.

3. In Chapter Ten, there is a script for a guided meditation to music on healing the inner child. This meditation is a moving, beautiful experience for most people at the workshops I conduct. It is loving, gentle, and healing, but may still bring up painful feelings for some people because it reminds them of the love that was lacking in their childhood. The inner child still needs to grieve over what was lost. If we don't complete the grieving process that empties out old pain, there isn't room for healing. As always, our inner work has proper times and seasons. After you read the meditation through, you can decide whether or not it feels right for you to do at this time in your life. You can then either tape the script to the suggested music or other music that comes to mind, or you may order the meditation with me as your guide.

PART TWO

Spiritual Beginnings

In the secret recesses of the heart
beyond the teachings of this world
calls a still, small voice
singing a song unchanged
from the foundation of the world.
Speak to me in sunsets and in starlight
Speak to me in the eyes of a child
You Who call from a smile
My cosmic beloved
Tell me who I am
And who I always will be.
Help me to remember.

—J. B.

CHAPTER FIVE

Who Am I?

Do you still have your high school yearbook? I do, and when I look at my picture it's still me all right—although I've gone through many metamorphoses in the years since I posed in that black turtleneck jersey, hair long and straight, trying my best to project the image of a carefully cultured young rebel who listened to Bach and read Beat poetry. My earrings, long and dangling, were the true sign of the counterculture. I knew I'd made it when Mr. Rinaldi, the housemaster of my high school class, called me into his office. "What happened to you? What's wrong? You don't set your hair anymore. And those earrings!" He rolled back his eyes and clapped his hand to his head just the way my mother had done that very same morning.

How many identities do we assume in the course of a lifetime? How many personalities form and dissolve like clouds in the sky? And yet the birth and death of each one seems like deadly serious business. We look for the ultimate one—the final statement of our being—forgetting that the waves of change will ultimately wash away each new sand castle. For who other than a dead person does not change? Who, in reality, is not made new in each moment? When our son Justin graduated from high school, he pored over books of poetry, quotes from famous people, and the lyrics of popular songs trying to find the perfect expression of his being to leave for posterity in the yearbook. So did each of his friends. Underneath the picture of a particularly winsome-looking, dark-haired girl I found the following quote:

When I was so young it seemed that life was so
wonderful, a miracle, it was beautiful, magical.
But then they sent me away to teach me how to be
sensible, logical, responsible, practical.
Won't you please tell me what we've learned?
I know it sounds absurd, but please tell me
who I am.

I thought about this young stranger, poised at childhood's end, who stared out from the yearbook pages. Her quote expressed the age-old longing of every human soul to feel the continual newness of the Natural Child, even as it discovers its expression in the unique personality that develops throughout our lifetime. Her words seemed so poignant to me, such an expression of our heartfelt search to find ourselves, that I copied out the quote and showed it to my husband, Myrin. He looked it over, smiled in sudden recognition and started fitting the first four lines to music that was popular a few years ago. He sang, "It was beautiful, magical . . . responsible, practical." I did remember, marveling at the ability of songwriters to distill the human condition in so few lines.

Finding out who we are is not an academic inquiry into the ultimate meaning of life. It's the very process of life, the blood and bones of the thoughts, feelings, and actions that make up each day. As long as we're prisoners of guilt, we cannot discover who we are, because the Natural Child is asleep, and our vitality is low. Bound by the chains of counterfeit conditional love that mortgages our souls to other people's opinions and expectations, we are too busy with all the masks, the false personalities, the people-pleasing, and the addiction to perfection to really live each moment as it happens. Instead, we want to control each moment and make sure that nothing upsets the apples so carefully arranged in our carts.

In case you haven't noticed, being the director of the universe and the controller of every interaction is no fun whatsoever. "Control freaks" have a dry, fearful, and self-righteous lifestyle. And since most people resent being controlled, personal relationships also suffer. When we feel helpless, the natural reaction is to grab for control as a cover-up for impotence and fear. But real power is found not in dictating the flow of events, but in having the flexibility to redirect our course to go with the ever-changing flow of possibilities that the universe unfolds before us.

The more we are constricted by our unhealthy guilt, the less we are able to notice how the flow is changing. *Guilt clogs our intuition* (the awareness of the flow), which normally can sense a subtle level of information in emotions, dreams, images, hunches, "coincidences," and the seemingly ordinary business of life. Intuitive information maximizes our creativity and allows us to assume roles not as creators and controllers of the universe, but as willing cocreators who mold the raw materials that a Higher Power provides.

Sometimes we control ourselves rigidly and pay the penalties of guilt in this life in the strange hope that our fear and repression will be considered "goodness" and buy us a spot in heaven. In other words, we may be miserable now, but we'll certainly get our reward later! A Jewish tzaddik, or wiseman, once gave a pupil sound advice. "When you die and get to heaven, God isn't going to ask you why you weren't as brave as Moses or as wise as Solomon. He's only going to ask you why you weren't yourself." And what are you going to say then? It was because my mother wanted me to be a doctor, or I was afraid to make my wife angry, or I thought you *liked* people with pursed lips and serious expressions, or someone told me that having a good time was a sin? Guilt is likely to seem very silly at the last trump, don't you think?

THE MANY ME'S

Roberto Assagioli, the Italian psychiatrist who developed psychosynthesis, pointed out that each one of us has a whole harem of personalities that live together under the auspices of the "I" we call me. We are often much more aware of some of our component parts—what Assagioli called *subpersonalities*—than we are of others. Take Joanne, a prim and tailored lawyer who came to a Mind/Body group. In her dreams she sported red silk lingerie straight out of the Frederick's of Hollywood catalog. Her sensual subpersonality is submerged in her shadow and comes to consciousness largely in dreams, but it is nonetheless part of her, along with the well-organized lawyer, the generous lady who serves Sunday dinner at the shelter for the homeless and the frightened little girl who's terribly afraid of rejection and has just gotten engaged for the first time at forty. In this maze of shadow, mask, and consciously chosen roles, who is the *real* Joanne?

We can shed some light on the answer to this question by looking at the interesting phenomenon called multiple personality disorder. Consider the hypothetical case of Marsha. It is 3:30 P.M. on Wednesday, and Marsha is just coming home from the hospital where she works as a nurse on the neonatal intensive care unit. She takes off and folds her work clothes carefully, puts on a pair of jeans, and settles down to watch a soap opera on television. Taking a long stretch, Marsha closes her eyes and yawns. A minute later, a sly smile begins to play around the corners of her mouth, and she goes back to her bedroom where she starts rummaging through the drawers until she finds her old rag doll, Sally. Holding the doll close, Betty, as she now calls herself, proceeds to the kitchen, where she makes Sally and herself a dinner of milk, cookies, and ice cream. Afterward, she and Sally fall asleep on her bed. When the phone rings at seven, Marsha is completely confused. Instead of meeting her date at six o'clock, she had another one of those strange blackouts, and *how* did that old doll get out of the drawer?

Multiple personality disorder is so compelling that it makes us rethink some of our most cherished assumptions. I can recall watching *The Three Faces of Eve* many years ago and marveling that three personalities, each as different from the others as day from night, could inhabit one body. Each personality was capable of controlling the gestures, the voice quality, the mind and memory, and even the body's physiology exclusively. We know that the mind has a profound influence on the body and that a change of attitude can change our hormones, cardiovascular system, respiratory system, and immune system, that it can indeed affect every cell and tissue. Nonetheless, it is incredible that one personality can be allergic, need glasses, or even have non–insulin dependent diabetes while the others don't! Furthermore, one personality may have a normal IQ while another is a genius. One may practice medicine, another may be an artist, while yet another may know languages unknown to the rest.

Only a decade ago, multiple personality disorder was considered rare, an anomaly, and some people believed that it didn't really exist. Now we know that it is fairly common, and that it develops in abused children who actually "split off" or dissociate new personalities to take the abuse while their original personality hides in the wings of consciousness. With time, a whole cadre of personalities may form, each capable of taking care of different aspects of life—each with another role, and each believing it is "who the person is." This is an extreme example of forming "false selves" as the result of emotional trauma and physical abuse.

In the case of a person who develops unhealthy guilt, the less severe but still very frightening childhood experience of conditional love results in the splitting off of false personalities or masks to please the parent and the splitting off of "unacceptable" personalities into the shadow. Sexuality is common shadow material, as it was with Joanne, but that doesn't mean that it stops exerting an influence. It only means that it cannot exert its normal, healthy influence. In 1987 and 1988, televangelists Jim Bakker and Jimmy Swaggart both fell victim to natural sexual impulses that had become damaged while composting in the bag of the shadow. While both condemned sexuality publicly, their repressed impulses surfaced in secret sexual liaisons. The unexplored shadow can be every bit as dangerous as one of the alter egos of a multiple personality. Although the shadow doesn't consciously control behavior and physiology, it does so unconsciously. And how can we change what we are unaware of?

The therapy for multiple personality disorder is aimed at reintegrating all the separate selves into one functional whole, under the auspices of a single personality. This means, of course, that most of the personalities—like Marsha's Betty—will have to disappear. What does it mean for a personality to disappear, to lose its memories and dreams, its past and its future—to lose its consciousness? Isn't this what we fear the most at death? The dissolution of the ego, the letting go of who we think we are, seems terribly frightening. But therapists who have watched this process in multiple personalities have discovered an amazing fact. Since none of the personalities is "real," none of them actually "dies." Just as we continue to be ourselves if we stop practicing our profession or get married or divorced, there is a core to all of us that is deeper than the endless personalities that we project like movies on a screen.

In 1974, Dr. Ralph Allison first described an ego state potentially present in all people with multiple personalities; he dubbed it the Inner Self-Helper. *The Inner Self-Helper claims not to have been formed at any specific time or for any reason, as were the others, but to have been with the person since birth.* It is characterized by love and goodwill, often describes itself as a conduit for God's love, and sometimes calls on a Higher Power for help. Rather than seeking to "take over" the body, as do the other personalities, it wants only to become one with them. This personality can be a great help to the therapist, pointing out mistakes in the therapy and making suggestions that help in the process of reintegrating the disparate personalities back into a functional whole.

The Inner Self-Helper bears a striking resemblance to the core Divinity within each person—the dyad comprised of the personal expression of Divine Consciousness that is our unique soul (the Natural Child) and the impersonal consciousness of Spirit (the Self) that enlivens the soul as electricity illuminates a light bulb. No matter how many slides we project, how many different false personalities we form, by themselves they have no life and no reality. While the experiences that we have in these false personalities add to our store of soul wisdom, the personalities themselves are not essential to who we are. Without the light of the Self, they are lifeless and dead. We may give these personalities up voluntarily, like the beatnik me that lasted only through the beginning of college, or we may struggle as some of the multiple personalities do, insisting that the personality is who we are.

The psychospiritual work of a lifetime is twofold. First, we must become aware of our different personalities—those in the light as well as those in the shadow—so that we can walk through life as a whole person without waging the kind of inner wars that Joanne was fighting. This is called psychological integration and wholeness. We have met our shadow, accepted our various parts, and learned to function as a coordinated being using all the different parts of our personality. Second, we need to recognize that even this well-integrated personality that we call me —formed to serve our needs and acting as a vehicle through which we can experience life and express the potential within us—is still not who we really are. It is not the essential Self/Soul unit or center that is with us from birth and that (as we'll see in the next chapter) appears to accompany us after bodily death.

When we experience ourselves as this essential center organized around the Self, rather than as any one of our roles, we can function optimally, unimpeded by fears and desires—as the apostle Paul described it, "in the world, but not of it." Self-realization has also been called enlightenment because it ends the illusion of faulty identification with our ego roles and awakens us to a more basic, enduring identity in which we feel safe, secure, loved, and capable of radiating these qualities to other people. In Self-realization, our personality—our ego—is seen as no more and no less important than the identity we have chosen to accomplish our unique work in the world. It's great to have a personality, all right, but it is no more "us" than the clothes we hang over the back of our chair when we go to bed at night.

THE I THAT DOESN'T CHANGE

In spite of the parade of ever-changing personalities that we have believed was us and regardless of all the changes—the successes and failures, the gains and the losses, the long dangling earrings and the little gold hoops, sickness and health, the brown, black, or blond hairs and the gray ones, the relationships come and gone—can we not recognize the same consciousness at our core as when we were young?

Stop for a moment *and go get a photograph of yourself when you were a child, preferably two or three years old. Look at that sweet little person, or imagine yourself at that age if you can't find a picture. It is still you, isn't it? You can still feel yourself in your bones, can't you? Different body, different experiences, same core. (If you've found a picture, hang it up somewhere—on the bathroom mirror or the refrigerator door, or in your meditation space, if you have one—where you will see it. This will help you remember and love your inner child.)*

We all know that the Natural Child—the joyful young soul that directly reflects the energy of the Self—doesn't have to do anything or be any particular way to feel good about herself. As in the multiple personality, that Inner Self-Helper has no attachment to being any particular way. No investment in any ego state. And frequently, as little children, we are in our core, our center, expressing the Natural Child directly without needing to filter it through a subpersonality or mask. This is exuberance, the enthusiasm or "possession by God" that makes children so healing to be around.

As we get older, we develop more and more subpersonalities and spend progressively more time in them of necessity. After all, if you're sitting at a word processor, as I am right now, you'd better be in the subpersonality called writer since Natural Child without a filter would be whooping it up and making patterns all over the page! We need our egos to perform certain functions. But if the filter gets too thick—if the ego state takes itself too seriously and begins to live as if its role were to glorify itself rather than to perform its appointed task—then the energy of the Self, the projector bulb, the Source of life that enlivens all our different ego states, can't get through. We then feel depressed and lacking in vitality.

SEARCHING FOR THE SELF: THE HERO'S JOURNEY

The search for the Self has been immortalized in myths and fairy tales of all cultures, in religious metaphor, and in cinema. Mythologist Joseph Campbell has called the search for Self the hero's journey. In his epic and scholarly book *The Hero with a Thousand Faces,* Campbell traces the evolution of human consciousness from the instinctual world of animal survival to the arena of shared experience, or compassion. Each one of us eventually makes this journey, venturing forth from the world of our temporal concerns into a spiritual realm apart from everyday life—the Kingdom of God, Heaven, Luke Skywalker's meeting with Yoda, the Grail Castle, the Underworld, the Dreamworld. During our adventures in this realm, we realize some deeper truth, some greater connection to the Source or Ground of our being. We then return to the temporal world transformed, capable of living our lives authentically, or as Nietzsche put it, like "a wheel rolling from its own center."

We are born with an instinct to make the journey, a deep knowledge that the temporal world is but a limited sphere of experience, a stage upon which far greater energies play. The metaphor that the philosopher Schopenhauer used was of human life as a dream in which we are unaware of the dreamer. Children are naturally attuned to a larger sphere of consciousness, to the invisible or noetic realm, as well as to the material world of temporal experience. We can learn a lot by listening to them. When our niece Alexa was six, we were riding together in the car one hot July day in a companionable silence. She suddenly announced in a matter of fact way and out of the blue that she loves words because sometimes when she hears them she knows whole stories about them from someplace long ago, someplace "beyond the world."

Jung talked about this knowledge beyond words, these stories in our bones, as archetypes or organizing patterns of human experience that are part of every person's consciousness at birth. They are the heritage of universal wisdom that resides in the Self—an instinctual pattern that reveals the path of return—the way to Self-realization and reunion with our Source.

We instinctively cheer for the hero who reaches beyond the pains and pleasures of this world and plumbs the mystery of life, returning from his journey to inspire us to do likewise. A few years ago, moviegoers thrilled to the hero archetype of young Luke Skywalker being tutored in the use of The Force by the esoteric master Yoda. The story of Jesus has likewise thrilled generations of humankind because it evokes the same archetype. Jesus assured us that he had come to show us The Way by which each of us could follow the path back to God and enter the Kingdom, just as he had. The Buddha, too, left detailed instructions about how we could realize the Self, as did many Hindu teachers and Kabbalistic rabbis writing as early as the first century.

PSYCHOSPIRITUAL ASPECTS OF MYTH AND SYMBOL

It is heartening that the lifescripts we act out in the hero's journey of the soul rediscovering its Source have been lived before. Myths, for example—those old stories whose very name is paradoxically synonymous with "untruth"—are actually hidden repositories of wisdom. In them, each character represents some part of ourselves, for ultimately the journey is an inward one, although it is often informed and aided by outside sources. The search for the Self is both a psychological and a spiritual journey. I know people who have meditated and sought esoteric wisdom for years, to no avail, because their temporal natures and the wiles of the ego have gone unexplored. Conversely, many people are psychologically self-astute but unschooled in directing attention to the spiritual realm.

Myths and fairy tales attune us to both the psychological and the spiritual. In studying them, we can forewarn ourselves of what we are likely to encounter within both the personal realm of our own psyches and the noetic realm of greater forces. We can take heart when we have reached the darkest point of the journey because we know from the stories of those who have gone before us that the dawn is at hand. And we can have faith that although we may seem to be following a narrow and perilous road alone, it has been tread countless times before. We are not now, nor will we ever be, alone.

The well-loved fable of Snow White, for example, is much more than a simple story. It is an archetypal psychological myth about healing the wounded child. By identifying with Snow White's experience, we are shown how to reunite the mask and shadow and recover the vitality of the Natural Child. We are also warned of the pitfalls along the way. I think of Snow White as the archetype of the "perfect" child who must overcome her false selves, face the wiles of her ego in the person of her wicked stepmother, and come face to face with death before she awakens to a realization of who she really is. Let's take a closer look at the outline and then some of the details of her story. Remember that in myths, as in dreams, every character represents a part of ourselves. Snow White and the wicked stepmother are one person, mask and shadow respectively.

The fairy tale takes us from the pain of total identification with the false self (the Wicked Queen who always needs to be "the fairest in the land"), through a life-and-death battle with the Natural Child (Snow White) who embodies the soul's desire to awaken and realize the Self.

The time of self-reflection and introspection necessary for realizing the Self is represented by Snow White's sojourn in the woods with the seven dwarfs. There, in the tiny woodland cabin, she struggles with the Wicked Queen's repeated attempts to kill her. The final phase of self-acceptance and love comes only when she is awakened by the handsome prince, who demonstrates the hero's act of compassion by joining in a relationship with her even though she appears dead.

During Snow White's time in the woods with the seven dwarfs, she repeatedly falls prey to her shadow, just as we all do in the process of psychological growth. The Wicked Queen (the shadow) visits her three times at the dwarfs' little cottage. Three times Snow White fails to recognize her stepmother despite the dwarfs' warnings to be on the lookout. Twice the dwarfs save Snow White, once from a corset that has been laced tight enough to strangle her, and a second time from a poison comb. Like all of us, Snow White knows her weak points but continues to succumb to them nonetheless until she is nearly destroyed.

On the Wicked Queen's third visit, Snow White swallows a bit of poisoned apple and dies, hitting the psychological bottom that is called the soul's dark night. But since the death is symbolic—the dark before the dawn—her body doesn't rot. In her prolonged sleep, the egodeath, she is actually reorganizing a new personality centered around the Self. But none of us makes it entirely alone. The final steps of integration require an act of grace, represented by the compassion of the Prince, who can see beyond the mask of death into her soul, an act of vision represented by the glass coffin in which she is enshrined. In his love, he carries the coffin away, and, when they hit a bump, the apple is dislodged and Snow White is reborn.

Theodor Seifert, a Jungian analyst, wrote an elegantly beautiful exposition of this fairy tale called *Snow White: Life Almost Lost*. In the following passage, he writes of the Wicked Queen who stands before her magic mirror and asks the question, "Mirror, mirror, here I stand. Who is the fairest in all the land?" Seifert notes:

> Here begins the difficult task of perceiving one's own image and one's own self without the demand—in the sense of being competitive—of being unique, the best, the most outstanding. This is an especially important question because here *two principles meet head on that appear to exclude each other*: On the one hand, each of us is unique, an individual who has not yet existed previously, clearly different from all other persons. On the other, however, clearly different does not

> mean better, more beautiful, ahead of the competition, but rather simply other, unique, "just as I am," clearly differentiated from every other. Precisely when this uniqueness is not combined with haughtiness and pride, community is possible both with other persons and with the newness developing out of one's own soul. But if we base our uniqueness on the devaluation of other persons, we are taking an isolating attitude that destroys community. I am placing myself apart from the community with people because I reject being like them and instead always want to be better and more beautiful. This isolation leads to loneliness, then to anxiety, and finally to the ever greater need to be better and more outstanding. This is a vicious circle that leads to the collapse of healthy, natural community [pp. 75–76, italics added].

The crux of escaping from guilt's narcissism is recognizing that we are no better and no worse than anyone else. We may have different roles to play, but none of us is really our roles. I am reminded here of an old teaching tale about a "Lord's Club." Everyone who belongs must be a nobleman, and none of the members wants anyone of lesser rank on the premises. So they trade off performing such roles as doorman, cook, groom at the stable, and guest. Since they all know that they are lords, no one feels one-up or one-down on anybody else, and the situation is most enjoyable. This story reminds us to relate to the Self, the Divinity, that is equally present in each of us rather than to our apparent roles.

Our ability to relate to the Self in others follows from our own psychological healing. This is the sphere of compassion, a word meaning literally to *suffer with*, to leave the isolation of one's personal sphere and enter into the life of another. Joseph Campbell calls compassion the flower of psychospiritual growth. In Campbell's *Creative Mythology: The Masks of God*, he retells the Grail legend as written by the medieval poet Wolfram von Eschenberg. The Holy Grail, the Passover chalice that Jesus used at the Last Supper and that received his blood when he came down from the cross, is a powerful archetypal symbol of our ability to live an authentic life that culminates in the flowering of compassion.

> In Wolfram's Castle of the Grail, where Celtic, Oriental, alchemical and Christian features are combined in a communion ritual of unorthodox form and sense, the young hero's spiritual test is to forget himself, his ego and its goals, and to participate with sympathy in the anguish of another life.
>
> —Joseph Campbell, *Creative Mythology: The Masks of God* [p. 454]

Jesus was describing the same thing when he said that only in losing our lives shall we gain them. In *The Power of Myth*, Campbell calls the Grail:

> . . . that which is attained and realized by people who have lived their own lives. The Grail represents the fulfillment of the highest spiritual potentialities of the human consciousness. . . . The Grail becomes symbolic of an authentic life that is lived in terms of its own volition, in terms of its own impulse system, that carries itself *between* the pairs of opposites of good and bad, light and dark. One writer of the Grail legend starts his long epic poem with a short poem saying, "Every act has both good and evil results." Every act in life yields pairs of opposites in its results. The best we can do is lean toward the light, toward the harmonious relationships that come from compassion with suffering, from understanding the other person [p. 197].

Campbell is pointing to a profound psychospiritual nexus. *Compassion, which is the interpersonal bridge, is the union of the temporal and spiritual planes.* It is the place where Divinity enters human relationship, as we will consider together in Part Three. In compassion, we are fully present in the moment. We can enter the moment with another person, and we can also be compassionate to life itself—entering the magnificence of a sunset, the power of a storm, the greening of spring leaves. All such moments of compassionate immediacy bring us into the fullness of the Self.

NATURAL EXPERIENCES OF THE SELF: THE ENCHANTMENT OF THE HEART

Participation in life, saying yes to life, requires the immediacy of our attention—our awareness. Whenever we are attentively present, no matter what the activity, we experience the Self and its attributes of peace, wisdom, and compassion. Did you ever tune in on the moment when you awakened from deep, dreamless sleep, that moment of total peace and contentment before your mind begins to whir and rumble with plan and worry? What about the moment when you kick off your shoes, heave a sigh of relief, and sit down with a cup of coffee after running around for a few hours. Do you know what I mean? The mind stops. What about the times you spend laughing with a loved one, hugging someone you care for, or walking in the fragrant woods? These are the moments we cherish, moments when we are in touch with the Self.

One winter day, I shared such a "holy moment" with our son Justin, then twenty, and his friend Brian. My mother was nearing the end of her life and needed live-in care, so the three of us were moving some extra furniture out to Brian's truck to make a bedroom for her health aide. Although I hadn't known Brian well before, I was impressed by his intelligent, good-natured manner. We had begun to get acquainted that morning while Justin was out for a walk in the woods. After he returned, Justin and I were carrying a set of drawers down the hall while Brian loaded other items onto the truck. I told Justin how much I liked Brian, and, in his wisdom, he replied, "It's not just that Brian is smart either, Mom. It's that he really cares about other people. He's kind. That's why I like him so much."

The three of us stood in the driveway loading furniture onto the truck a few minutes later, joking and really enjoying one another's company. The February sun was unusually warm and seemed to enhance the comfortable feelings flowing between us. Suddenly time seemed to stop and we were suspended in a moment of transcendent peace, kindness, caring, and mutual positive regard. We shared an experience of the Self in which love flowed unobstructed across a three-way bridge that linked all of us to something greater. In that moment there was a completeness. Everything was all right with the world. We were fully present in the moment and with each other.

The Greek Orthodox priest Archimandrite Kallistos Ware calls the present "the point where time touches eternity." The time-bound world and the transcendent realm meet in these moments when we experience the Self. The noted psychologist Abraham Maslow called these "peak experiences." Colors seem unusually vivid, scents incredibly fragrant, sounds unusually rich, and textures almost alive. It is as though an invisible veil is lifted from the world, allowing its luminous beauty to shine forth clearly. There is no fear, only love, peace, wisdom, interconnectedness, and an overwhelming sense of love and safety that abide in the now.

The ancient philosophers compare the Self to a stone lying peacefully at the bottom of a pond. It is always there, but when the surface of the pond is disturbed, we cannot see it. The pond is a metaphor for the mind. When the mind is busy ruminating and worrying—the usual state of affairs—the Self remains hidden behind the mental storms. But when the mind quiets down, the stone is seen once more. The enjoyment of gardening or walking in nature comes because past and future fade away. Only the immediate connection to the earth and its beauty remain. The peaceful, loving quality of life's Source floods through our connection to the moment. "Ah, I love the woods," we think. But the peace is not inherent in the forest or the garden, the "beloved" that temporarily holds our attention. It is present within us. And when we connect to this inner wellspring, we feel our connection to all of life so much more strongly.

Literature and poetry abound with accounts of holy moments during which the Self and its connection to the Source are revealed and the soul stands witness in joy and awe. Literature and language professor Rhoda Orme-Johnson cites a variety of remarkable literary accounts of these transcendent moments. She quotes playwright Eugene Ionesco's *Present Past, Past Present*:

> Once, long ago, I was sometimes overcome by a sort of grace, a euphoria. It was as if, first of all, every notion, every reality was emptied of its content. After this emptiness . . . , it was as if I found myself suddenly at the center of pure ineffable existence. . . . I think that I became one with the one essential reality, when, along with an immense, serene joy, I was overcome by what I might call the stupefaction of being, the certainty of being. . . . I say that with words that can only disfigure, that cannot describe the light of this profound, total organic intuition which, surging up as it did from my deepest self, might well have inundated everything, covered everything, both my self and others.

These holy moments are what writer James Joyce called epiphanies—moments of stasis or profound stillness in which the mind is no longer disturbed by either desire or repulsion and simply stops. In Joyce's *Portrait of the Artist as a Young Man*, the character Stephen Daedelus comments that,

> The instant wherein that supreme quality of beauty, the clear radiance of the esthetic image, is apprehended luminously by the mind which has been arrested by its wholeness and fascinated by its harmony is the luminous silent stasis of esthetic pleasure, a spiritual state very like to that cardiac condition which the Italian physiologist Luigi Galvani, using a phrase almost as beautiful as Shelley's, called the enchantment of the heart.

LEARNING TO EXPERIENCE THE SELF

Glimpses of the Self occur intermittently and often by accident at times when thoughts slow down. But most of us are unable to feel peaceful, centered, and connected to the Self as a matter of choice because we have been taught little about how to use the most powerful tool we have—the mind. My sleepless patients know this well and usually complain about how the mind has a life of its own, particularly in the middle of the night! Many people take up the practice of meditation in the hopes of learning to "pull the plug" on the mind when it is chasing around fruitlessly, creating nothing but obsessive anxiety. In this state we are literally saying no to life because we are not present to experience it. We are trapped by the mind.

The ancient science of yoga, meaning *union* with the Self, is based on the knowledge, as is said in Patanjali's Yoga Sutras, that the "mind is as restless as the wind" and that the experience of the Self requires making the mind one's servant rather than letting it be our master. The mental and physical practices of yoga are therefore aimed at learning to quiet the mind and direct it in an orderly fashion. This does not mean languishing in a state of bliss and dropping out of the world. It means centering ourselves in the present so that we can perform our actions in the world with greater awareness: more honestly, lovingly, competently, and confidently.

Learning to use the mind as a tool, and *to think by choice* rather than in reaction to self-spun fantasies and reruns of old tapes, is what yoga is all about. When thinking is not required and the mind is allowed to rest, the Self is automatically experienced. Mental training is the cornerstone of many systems of martial arts, schools of meditation, and ancient philosophies that have appealed to only a slim segment of westerners. But during the last decade, techniques of mind/body control have reached the popular mainstream through psychology and medicine. Dr. Herbert Benson and others have demystified ancient yogic practices by exploring their underlying physiology, making them available as medical treatments for stress and anxiety-related illness regardless of one's religious or spiritual beliefs.

The beauty of these techniques, many of which are described and taught in detail in *Minding the Body, Mending the Mind*, is that they are compatible with any worldview, secular or religious, and form the basis of a science of mind. All of these practices were originally formulated as methods for accessing the Self, a side effect of which is a calming down of the fight-or-flight response. Many people nowadays begin to practice meditation or the physical postures of hatha yoga primarily for these physiological side effects, and then continue to practice them because they enjoy the experience of the Self and the benefits of increased psychological self-awareness that accompanies meditation.

BASIC MEDITATION

Anytime that you are in touch with the Self, rather than caught up in the isolating concerns of the ego, you are experiencing the meditative state. While this can happen naturally, if you have a more formal meditation practice that trains the mind to quiet down, the Self can be experienced more easily. Two basic schools of meditation have been handed down through the centuries. You can read in depth about their history, similarities, and differences in Daniel Goleman's *The Meditative Mind*. In *concentration meditation*, the mind is focused on a specific stimulus like a candle flame, a word, a prayer, a picture of a holy person, the breath, or anything that creates a single-minded focus. This process eventually results in an experience of the Self. In *mindfulness* or *open-focus meditation*, an attempt is made to fix the mind in the Self and then to observe the ever-changing flow of thoughts, emotions, sensations, and perceptions.

Concentration meditation is an ancient technique used in many spiritual traditions. It has been popularized most recently by transcendental meditation and explored scientifically by Dr. Herbert Benson, who called the specific bodily changes induced by concentration meditation the relaxation response. The idea is to keep the mind completely occupied with a specific, repetitive stimulus that derails it from its usual cares. From a physiological point of view, the particular stimulus makes no difference. You can elicit the relaxation response equally easily by mentally repeating the word "one" in time to every outbreath, or focusing on the sensation of the breath as it moves in and out of the belly or the nostrils, or focusing on a more spiritual stimulus. Since meditation arose as a spiritual practice meant to reunite the separated soul with the Divine Whole, a *mantra*—a name of God, a prayer, or some aspect of the Divine—was the preferred focus. In choosing a mantra, if this appeals to you, find an aspect of Divinity that you most naturally relate to.

A generic Sanskrit mantra that fits any religious tradition is the repetition of *Ham Sah*—*Ham* on the inbreath and *Sah* on the outbreath. *Ham* means "I am," and *Sah* means the "Self." The mantra is meant to remind us of who we really are, and the ancients believed that if you listened carefully to your breath it whispered your true identity to you every minute of your life. *Ham*, I Am, *Sah*, the Self. And, with practice, this mantra does repeat itself automatically—you find yourself listening to it rather than initiating it.

Jewish and Christian traditions likewise focus on concentration meditation. The Jewish mystics from the Kabbalistic tradition repeat the four Hebrew letters of the tetragrammaton—in English, YHVH—that were given by God for the Jews to use in lieu of His holy, unpronounceable name. Some Christian sects have taken these Hebrew letters and anglicized them to Jehovah, but in the Jewish tradition the letters are never pronounced together but are combined in a variety of ways as a focus for meditation that leads to a direct experience of God. Rabbi Aryeh Kaplan was a Jewish mystic and scholar who wrote several books on different aspects of Jewish mysticism and its practice, and *Jewish Meditation*, referenced in the reading list, is a good beginning if you are interested in this tradition.

The Christian meditation tradition is also very rich. The desert fathers, early Christian monks who lived during the fourth century, lived a life of contemplative prayer focusing on the mantra known as the prayer of the publican: "Lord Jesus Christ, Son of God, have mercy upon me, a poor sinner." The short form of this "Jesus prayer" in its original Greek is *Kyrie Eleison*, or "Lord, Have Mercy."

Bill was sixty when I met him at the Mind/Body Clinic early one spring as the Boston snows were beginning to melt. A tall, lanky man with a big smile and the callused hands of a laborer, Bill had a chronic form of leukemia that had been stable for several years, but that was beginning to worsen. Bill's interest in meditation was threefold. He thought it would help him with the discomforts of cancer treatment, that it might possibly slow down the illness, and that it would help him strengthen his connection to God. And meditation is truly such a gift. The eighteenth-century Jewish tzaddik Rabbi Nachman compared meditation to a tree whose fruits we can eat in this life and whose roots remain to nourish us in the time beyond.

When we talked about choosing a mantra, Bill immediately thought of *Kyrie Eleison*. As we sat and meditated together, Bill mentally sang to himself "kyrie" on the inbreath and "eleison" on the outbreath. Within minutes, his tension evaporated, and the peace in the room was palpable. When he opened his eyes, filled with tears, Bill told me that, in those twenty minutes, his fear and loneliness had disappeared. He felt powerfully connected, in a way that words were inadequate to express, with all the people through all the centuries who had intoned that prayer of Jesus in their hearts. This is what we are told by the Hindus, Buddhists, Christians, Jews, Sufis, and others for whom meditation is a living spiritual connection—that the old mantras are infused with the love and faith of all those who have uttered them before, that they are a kind of living talisman containing the collective power of many hearts' longing for reunion with their Source. For this reason, choosing an "established" mantra from an ongoing spiritual tradition is often more powerfully centering than inventing a new mantra.

The steps for concentration meditation, explained by Benson in *The Relaxation Response* and described at length in *Minding the Body, Mending the Mind*, are simple:

1. Sit or lie down with your spine straight and your body balanced and symmetrical (in other words, with uncrossed arms and legs).

2. Relax your muscles as best you can, either by stretching briefly or mentally checking your body from head to toe.

3. Focus on the mantra, repeating it in time to your breath.

4. If you get distracted, which you will, take a letting-go breath and return to the mantra.

The most important part of the process is *attitude*. The guilty notion that you should be able to concentrate perfectly and outwit your wandering mind after a few minutes, a few weeks, a few months, or even a few years of practice is self-defeating. Don't fall into the trap of judging the "quality" of the meditation at all. Just do it, taking heart in the words of St. Francis, who reassured us that even if the heart should wander for the whole hour of meditation, it is still an hour well spent.

One of the most powerful things that happens from the practice of meditation is that you gradually begin to understand that you are *not* your mind. Thoughts come and go, but you learn to sit and watch them like so many clouds passing across the sky. You are *having* thoughts, but you are *not* your thoughts. Sometimes, naturally, your mind will get carried away with thoughts, and temporarily you will identify with them. Then you notice, "Ah, thinking," and you take a breath or two and go back to your mantra or your breath, once again passively disregarding the passing thoughts and strengthening what I call the mental muscles of letting go.

The other great meditation tradition, called the path of insight, is associated with the Buddhist tradition. It begins with the practice of mindfulness, *sathipatthana*, or bare attention. The meditator begins by focusing on the breath as an attempt to become one with the Self or indwelling Spirit. In many languages, the word for breath is synonymous with Spirit. In Hebrew, *ruach* means breath, wind, and spirit. In Greek, *pneuma* means air, breath, or spirit. Our English word *respiration* likewise comes from the Latin root *spiro*, meaning breath or spirit.

Once centered in the breath, then, like a detective the meditator stays silently on the lookout for thoughts, feelings, and perceptions, just noticing his own immediate experience without judging it, commenting on it, or attempting to change it. After a while, the meditator begins to see that the cohesive view of reality he holds so dear is built up of successive units of "mind-stuff" that are in themselves meaningless, and an entirely new view of the mind is revealed, a process called the development of insight, or *vipassana*, which leads to the state of *nirvana* in which the mind and the objects it contemplates are experienced as one.

In either form of meditation, you will eventually learn to take up the position of watching or witnessing your thoughts rather than identifying with them. This is enormously empowering, because we are so often bullied and victimized by our own thoughts. As a technique of psychological growth, the ability to detach from the illusion that thoughts are reality is of tremendous benefit. Pretty soon you become aware that when your mind is not identified with the thoughts and you can let them pass by without judging them or embroidering on them, the basic consciousness we call Self automatically emerges, peacefully witnessing the antics of the mind. In some schools of meditation, in fact, the Self is called the Witness.

Stop for a moment and try witnessing your mind before you read on. Close your eyes and take a couple of nice, deep letting-go breaths, real sighs of relief. As you do so, let your body sink comfortably back in your chair, and let your breath find its own natural rhythm. Pause in the comfortable feeling of your breath. For the next minute, pretend you are a detective listening in on an important conversation, alert for every word or image that crosses your mind. With a relaxed yet keenly interested attitude, eavesdrop closely on your mind as you stay centered in your breathing. Continue for a minute or two.

What happened? Perhaps you started to witness your thoughts arising and fading away, but then a particularly juicy one popped up and you got all wrapped up in it. We do that all the time, of course, identifying totally with the mind-movie, the dream, of the moment. Or maybe you sat quietly by the metaphoric river of your mind, just letting the thoughts float past while staying peacefully centered in your witness. Or, will wonders never cease, perhaps your chatterbox of a mind actually rested for a change!

About half the people who try witnessing for the first time come up empty-handed and quite surprised. Where did all the thoughts go? Steve Maurer, current director of the Mind/Body Clinic, often jokes that the mind gets embarrassed when you watch it. When the mind quiets down, people report feeling a pleasant, relaxed peacefulness that often intensifies to a sense of loving connectedness with life. When you are witnessing, you have stepped back out of the mind into the Self's essential nature, which is peace and love. You have temporarily corrected the case of mistaken identity and remembered who you really are.

If you have been practicing loving your inner child, you are probably acquainted with how wonderful the current of love feels as your whole nervous system and every cell in your body responds to your imagination. This is similar, but less intense, than the feeling you will eventually get as you learn to disengage from the stream of thinking that pulls you out of your center. We have all had different experiences of this deeply restful, perfectly loved and loving state. I remember feeling that way when I would sit in silence and watch my boys sleep when they were infants. Only this time you are watching your own Self, remembering the same wellspring of love that we cherish in children and worship in nature, the Source that dwells within us as our own essential nature.

During the day, when your ego jumps in and starts judging and criticizing you, try taking a few breaths and moving out of your mind into the position of the witness. You can do this by comforting the inner child and then letting the image go, and resting in the peaceful, centered feelings that remain. Or you may be able to step directly into the witness by becoming the watcher of your thoughts, as we just practiced. The technique doesn't matter—do what is most natural for you. After a dose of love, a moment of connection with who you really are, the conditioned pull of your ego that is always advertising your "limitations" will seem much weaker.

I like to begin my own meditation practice by centering in the Self, by remembering a holy moment and then concentrating on the current of love and connectedness that remains after the memory has faded. If you practice remembering the Self, whether in meditation or throughout the day, you will slowly but surely begin to honor your own worthiness *because you will experience it directly*. You will know without needing to think about it that you are not your fear, your desires, your anger, your limitations. These are only states of mind. Correcting the case of mistaken identity, you will realize that you are your Self.

THE POWER OF RITUAL CENTERING

Most of us are so busy with the external necessities of life that our attention is constantly scattered, jumping from one thing to the next. Life necessitates giving our energy to many different roles. In just the last twenty-four hours of activities and relationships, for example, I've been mother, wife, friend, daughter, sister-in-law, cook, cleaner, party-goer, meditator, sleeper, and writer. We identify with some of our roles very strongly, and, when we do we are more likely than ever to forget the Self. But any activity, when conducted with awareness, can connect us to the Self. Washing dishes is no less of an invitation to a holy moment than is a sunset. Listening to friends, playing with children, frolicking with pets, sharing from the heart, meditating—these are ways that we naturally center. But whenever we do centering activities as a regular practice—with the intention of strengthening our connection to the Source—we are making use of the tremendous power of ritual.

Meditation, for instance, is a ritual whose purpose is remembering the Self. In doing it daily, we make a commitment to a vision—to a purpose for life—that has real power to bring about change. By putting time and energy aside to remember the Self, we bring it into our consciousness. And, as we'll see in the next chapter, our longing to return to the Source, to remember the Self, is also one way that we attract grace.

Meditation, however, is a solitary ritual. There are also communal rituals that serve as important reminders that we are all players in a great, repeating drama. Such rituals help prevent some of the suffering that comes from taking ourselves too seriously, thinking that we are something special (thinking that we are especially good and assuming that we are especially bad are equally troublesome attitudes). The problem with "special" is that it implies "different from." Since the Self—the common core of consciousness—is of equal value in every person, we continue to be imprisoned by our egos and to suffer from guilt as long as we insist on specialness. In ritual—a communal act repeated in the same way throughout history—we lose our individual illusion of specialness and enter a group identity in which the Self can more easily emerge.

In the Jewish family, on the eighth day of a male child's life there has traditionally been a ceremony called a bris—the ritual circumcision—to signify the child's entrance into the ancient covenant with God. The family gathers to share a new bonding, in the moment of the child's pain, which quickly gives way to the celebration of life. The ceremony is a salute to the promise of the newborn, to the continuity of the family, to a cultural tradition that lasted through a vast diaspora as Jews were scattered over the face of the earth, to a spiritual heritage reaching back through the millenia to the moment when Moses received the tablets on Sinai. In Catholicism, there is the sacrament of communion, the mystery of becoming one with the body and blood—the vision and Spirit—of Jesus, which he gave us as a perpetual reminder of life's purpose and his ever-present love and forgiveness. And, in both Judaism and Christianity, there is the ritual of keeping the Sabbath—putting aside one day a week—to remember and to center.

There is power in such rituals when they are performed consciously, with the understanding that they are acts of centering, because they were designed to align the individual with something larger—family, tribe, culture, God. At the moment of alignment, all the pieces fall into place like the colored glass in a kaleidoscope. Everything is centered, the pattern is whole, and we are in our appointed places, connected by invisible threads to a greater wholeness. We live for a moment in seamless, sacred time, and we know who we are and where we are. The players in the drama are all arranged according to plan, and everything is right with the world.

Every culture, every tradition, has rituals that mark life's passages and allow its members to recenter periodically and make sure they are on the proper path. Some cultures, like that of the Native Americans, had sacred geographical spaces called the mesas, mountaintops where rituals of centering were traditionally performed. Most religions have adopted enclosures—temples and churches originally built according to a sacred geometry that was intended to line up invisible force fields felt by mystics and recorded in the universal language of mathematics and geometry. The human heart is likewise a sacred place. And, if we develop the ritual of entering it each day in prayer, meditation, or just a moment of silent gratitude, we will find ourselves realigned with a Higher Power, the force of creative love, wisdom, humor, and intuition that will guide us along the hero's journey.

DREAMS AND INTUITION

Although we may not consciously know what roles and archetypes we are acting and enacting in our journeys, our unconscious knows and tries to communicate that information in reverie, daydreams, unbidden insights, and the nightly unfolding of our dreams. We spend approximately one third of life asleep, and each one of us dreams about 20 percent of that time. Laboratory studies reveal that we enter REM (rapid eye movement) sleep four to five times a night. Dreams always accompany REM sleep whether we remember them or not, and, if we pay attention, our dreams provide a vast storehouse of creative inspiration, psychological understanding, and spiritual direction.

The literature on dreams abounds with anecdotes on creative insights and invention:

> Descartes first formulated the basic philosophical stance of Rational Empiricism which undergirds the entire development of modern science as the result of a vivid dream experience. Kekulé, who was inspired to understand that the molecular structure of benzene is ring-shaped as a result of dreaming of a snake biting its tail, once admonished his colleagues in basic research: "Gentlemen, learn to dream!" Albert Einstein, when asked late in his life just when and where the idea of the Theory of Relativity had first occurred to him, replied that he could not trace the earliest intimations any further than a dream he had had in adolescence. He recounted that in his dream he was riding on a sled. As the sled accelerated, going faster and faster until it approached the speed of light, the stars began to distort into amazing patterns and colors, dazzling him with the beauty and power of their transformation. He concluded by saying that in many ways, his entire scientific career could be seen as an extended meditation on that dream.
>
> —Jeremy Taylor, *Dreamwork* [pp. 6–7]

Jeremy Taylor is a Unitarian minister and psychologist who has been leading dream groups for more than twenty years. In my opinion, his book *Dreamwork* is the single best exploration of the psychospiritual meaning of dreams ever written. He sums up the heart of dreamwork as follows:

> Dreams come always in the service of promoting wholeness. They have an inherently opening effect, always bringing to consciousness those aspects of our own being which we have closed out of our waking experience. . . . Even the worst nightmare has as one major reason for its existence the correction of some imbalance in waking perception, attitude or behavior [pp. 18, 45].

Freud called dreams the "royal road" to the unconscious. They come in service of promoting awareness, often presenting us with information we have tried to deny. Part of my own ongoing recovery from guilt involved the admission that I am an adult child of an alcoholic with my own addictions to guilt, codependent behavior, and workaholism. Because the alcohol use in my family of origin was covert and the family seemed quite functional, I never thought of addiction and codependency as issues that affected me personally. This kind of denial is quite common in adult children of alcoholics.

My denial was broken by a clever play on words in a very vivid, attention-getting dream. In the dream, my mother and I are floating on a raft in the deep end of a large swimming pool. I swim to the other end where several old women are gathered. One is in her nineties and is obviously a woman of great spiritual wisdom. I want to introduce her to my mother so she can share her wisdom with us so I excitedly swim back to the raft to tell my mother. By the time I get back to the wisdom woman, I find her lying close to death by the edge of the pool. Her chest has been opened and the meat carved off like the breast of a turkey. The other women in the pool are eating sandwiches of her meat. I am incensed, disappointed, and bewildered. "Why didn't you open a can of tunafish?" I scream. "We prefer cold turkey sandwiches" is the terse answer.

I awakened perplexed and disturbed—a good sign that dream contents are particularly relevant. In the twilight phase of half-wakefulness, as I lay rerunning the dream and committing it to memory so that I could record it in my dream journal, I didn't catch the pun of "cold turkey," since the unconscious is quite literal. When fully awakened and writing down the dream, however, the colloquial meaning of "cold turkey" jumped out at me, and I couldn't help receiving the wisdom woman's advice with a gale of laughter that broke right through my denial. It was time to own up to and recover from the addictions that had kept me a prisoner for so long before they literally killed me. It was time to go cold turkey.

The first step to recovery from any behavior pattern is awareness, and awareness of our ongoing family addiction pattern was the true gift of the dream. Apparently in order to make sure I got the message, my sleep during the next three weeks was filled with addiction dreams of two sorts. The first were what I think of as typical dreams filled with metaphor and many levels of symbolism; the second were what I think of as instructional dreams from the realm of the Higher Self. The latter category is not a dream per se, but a series of illuminating explanations that one hears without visual accompaniment.

Dreams are also an excellent source of information about the shadow. Dreams in which we are being pursued or attacked often represent the split of the psyche into its parts, revealing the inner wars in which dark shadow figures threaten to destroy the ego masks we have adopted to replace the reality of who we are. In a dream, all the characters, even the scary ones, represent some aspect of ourselves. A woman at one of my workshops, who had been recording and working with her dreams for years, told of a very interesting shadow dream in which she is a midwife attending the birth of two babies. The first mother has a healthy, chubby infant. The second birth is long and slow, and the baby presents breech, feet first. With disgust, she realizes that the baby's legs end in cloven hooves and that she is assisting the birth of a demon. As the dream ends, she already understands that the dream refers to the work she has done in becoming herself, in giving birth to herself. She has developed a healthy ego, and she has also been resolute in seeking out and facing her shadow, which seems "almost born" to her. When it is fully born, she thinks, and can stand alongside the pink, chubby baby, then she will be whole. She awakens feeling strong and peaceful.

You may have already found different levels of symbolism in the dreams we have just shared. Taylor's experience, and my own, is that there are multiple levels of meaning to every dream and that new levels of meaning appear as the dreamer goes through various life passages and continues to grow and change. This is quite obvious and delightful if you keep a dream journal and review the dreams periodically. Edgar Cayce, Jeremy Taylor, and other dream experts counsel the dreamer to think the dream through and try to get it settled in memory before moving around in bed. Even if you can catch a tiny dream fragment and lay still with it, more of the dream is likely to come. Record the dream in the present tense, which also aids recall, and then choose a title evocative of the dream's content. For example, I call my addiction dream Cold Turkey. The woman at the workshop called her shadow dream Birth into Wholeness. If you keep your dream journal by your bed, with the intent of recording dreams either as they occur in the night or in the morning upon awakening, your dream recall will increase substantially.

In addition to creative and psychological insights, dreams have long been regarded as messengers from the spiritual realm. As such, they speak the language of the Higher Self—the universal language of myth and symbolism that stays constant across all cultures and all times. Jeremy Taylor reminds us that:

> Myth and dream stem from the same ultimate source in the collective unconscious, and it is possible to understand myth as "collective

> dreams"—collective expressions of dramas that are universally human and thus are always experienced as personal, while at the same time they can be seen as repeating themselves endlessly in the individual and collective lives and dramas of all human beings.
>
> —*Dreamwork* [p. 72]

Since myth and dream are both expressions of the collective unconscious, ancient archetypes of spiritual growth often appear as dream motifs. These are as applicable now as they have been for thousands of years. They may inform the dreamer either about some current passage or an overall direction in life. Myrin and I had a shared dream about such a mythic archetype on the first night we spent together almost two decades ago. This short dream, like all dreams, is filled with layer upon layer of symbolism. In twenty years, we have unraveled many of its secrets, but it continues to reveal fresh insights to us. In the dream it is night. We are standing on top of a stone tower on a tiny, rocky island in the middle of the sea. The tower is struck by lightning, catches fire, and begins roaring like an inferno. Holding hands, we jump into the sea. Both of us awakened from the dream at the same moment. Hearts pounding, eyes wide, and still breathless from the vivid imagery, we turned to each other and said, "I just had the most amazing dream."

While neither Myrin nor I had even heard the word *archetype* at the time of what we called the Tower Dream, we both knew intuitively that the dream symbolized the ancient drama of death and rebirth, and that it was offering us psychological and spiritual insight into our new life together. The significance of the dream unfolded dramatically two years later when we were first introduced to the Tarot deck. Flipping through the deck, we spied a card called The Tower and were astounded when we recognized it as our shared dream.

> What the Tarot represents is an allegorical journey, each card being the experience of something (a universal energy) along the way, rather like the episodes in Dante's *Divine Comedy*, Bunyan's *Pilgrim's Progress* or even Tolkien's *Trilogy of the Ring*. . . . Esoteric tradition, as represented by the Tarot, makes some very basic statements about man and the nature of the Universe which is his ultimate environment. It says that there is a perfect order which one has the capacity to perceive, and that there is no such thing as an accident. For every movement of every leaf on every tree there is a reason, and every movement of every thing is inter-related. . . . The doctrine that our universe is so precisely ordered is basic to the Tarot, as is the idea

> that the Tarot images accurately symbolize the framework of the Universe.
>
> —Robert Wang, *Qabalistic Tarot* [pp. 4–6]

The Tower card is called the equilibrating path of the personality and represents the union of the intellect (the path of reason) and the intuition (the path of the heart). In most versions of the Tower card, the crown or capstone of the tower is struck off by lightning, symbolizing the abrupt destruction of those values and roles we had previously considered to constitute reality. At one level, the tower is symbolic of the ego, destroyed by the sudden force and power of the Higher Self that urges the individual along the journey to God consciousness. At another level, the tower represents belief systems, religions, or any constraining force, which, in our case, extended to previous marriages, relationships with parents, and spiritual values, to name but a few of the changes we suddenly found ourselves swimming through.

As the card revealed, our growth together has been through the balance of the intellect and the heart, occasional thunderbolts periodically burning down the tower of our individual and shared concepts and pushing us into new awarenesses. During the difficult times of upheaval that have ensued, the Tower Dream has always served as a touchstone to remind us of the path of partnership and growth that, for whatever reason, is ours to follow together. The dream has also been an important reminder that growth is often a painful process, but an orderly one, that has been summarized in many different ancient wisdom sources such as the Tarot. Jeremy Taylor explains that:

> The Tarot deck is clearly one concrete example of this archetypal tradition of "The Book of All Knowledge." There is a story that the Tarot deck was born in the imaginations of the last librarians of the great library at Alexandria as they watched the collected wisdom of the world disappear in flames during the Moslem invasion in 646 A.D. As they saw the library burn, they are said to have turned to one another and agreed that they must never allow the collected wisdom of the ages to be so easily lost again. They set about creating a set of images embodying the wisdom that had been lost in the fire—the archetypal patterns of knowledge of the collective unconscious. They fabricated these images and invented popular entertainments and games of skill and chance so that the uninitiated common people would love the deck and take it with them everywhere, dispersing it

over the face of the earth so that it could never be lost in such a fashion again.

—Dreamwork [p. 133]

Dreams are one more way that the Spirit gives us to develop our intuition and literally to recenter so that we stand in line with the flow rather than opposing it, an image that came to me very graphically in a dream. At one point in my life when I was wondering about the perennial question of free will versus destiny, I had the following dream. We are digging a pond in our back yard. The hole is eight or ten feet deep, and water is beginning to seep in. There is a large, tidal river in back of the house (there is no such river in fact) and, as the pond fills, water begins to redistribute in the series of marshes and canals that feed the river. Suddenly, the river changes its course and a tributary springs up in my neighbors' driveway, filling their cellar with water. I feel very guilty. Then I pick up the newspaper and read that geologists have predicted that the river is about to change its course. With great relief, I realize that I did not redirect the flow of the river, but was just the Universe's agent. When I reviewed this dream, one of its many levels of meaning had to do with the question I had posed to my Higher Self before sleep—the question of free will. The dream answered with a lovely metaphor reassuring me that I was not the Divine Director of the flow, but merely its agent and that my individual act fit into a larger plan. I have come to think of free will as the choice to become aware and use one's intellect and intuition to go with the flow and make the hero's journey, or to remain unaware and therefore oppose the flow, getting lost in the pitfalls that make the journey longer and harder.

Poets such as Kabir, Rabindranath Tagore, William Blake, Rainer Maria Rilke, Alfred Lord Tennyson, Walt Whitman, Kahlil Gibran, and the Old Testament poet who wrote the piercingly beautiful *Song of Solomon*, or the *Song of Songs*, have the gift of putting dream, myth, and metaphor into words that can awaken the reader and realign him with the flow. Take a few letting-go breaths and retire into the stillness of your heart before you read the following poem.

Be still
Listen to the stones of the wall
Be silent, they try
To speak your
Name.

Listen
To the living walls.
Who are you?
Who
Are you? Whose
Silence are you?

—Thomas Merton

SUGGESTIONS FOR THE READER

1. Can you remember times when you were spontaneously centered and in touch with the Self? These times are good touchstones—reminders for when you're feeling scattered, off-center, and identified with the ego. Try taking a couple of letting-go breaths and remembering one of these peak experiences, one of these holy moments.

2. Practice witnessing a few times each day. Each time you try it you will be building up new mental pathways for dealing with your guilty thoughts. *Remember that the witness position is your center—it is like the eye of the storm.* No matter what is happening, the witness always feels safe and connected to the Source of love. Witnessing is worth practicing.

3. Let a meditation practice develop naturally and spontaneously *if it feels good to you*. Otherwise put aside fifteen or twenty minutes daily to walk in nature, write a poem, listen to music, or engage in any activity that is a natural meditative experience. The key to meditation is to let it be a pleasure. If it becomes a "should" activity, you will experience your ego rather than your Self, and the guilty need no more practice at that!

4. Try recording your dreams every night. It helps to enter the next day's date and day of the week in your journal as your last act before retiring. Taylor also suggests that you write a concise line about why you want to remember your dreams. What is your purpose? Sharing your dreams with a person or persons who are respectful and interested in shared psychospiritual growth gives great depth to dreamwork. Should you choose to do so, consider these basic ground rules adapted from Taylor's *Dreamwork*:

a. Every dream comes in service of wholeness and healing.

b. Every dream has multiple levels of meaning.

c. It is unlikely that you will exhaust all the meanings in one session—or ever, for that matter.

d. Whenever you comment on another person's dream, use the language and understanding "If this were my dream" before you make your interpretation. The fireplug that represents male sexuality to you may or may not have that meaning for the other person. Even Freud said that sometimes a cigar is just a cigar! Although dreams contain universal archetypes at one level, they are psychological projections on another level. Any interpretation of someone else's dream is just that—a projection that may or may not be on target. Taylor makes the point that the only reliable touchstone for an interpretation is the little thrill of recognition, the chill of gooseflesh, that lets you know your intuition is working. It is up to the dreamer to let others know whether or not a certain interpretation is on the mark.

e. Make the sharing safe and agree on ground rules such as anonymity, which means that the dreams can be discussed outside the group context, but only in such a way that the individual dreamer cannot be identified. At times, a certain member may also ask for strict confidentiality that forbids the dream to be shared in any way.

CHAPTER SIX

Spiritual ReVision: A Nation of Closet Mystics

I can still remember being seven years old and coming back from the first day of Sunday school at the conservative temple my family attended. The entire way home in the bus, surrounded by schoolmates, I was unusually quiet and lost in fantasy. The exotic and beautiful curves of the Hebrew alphabet filled me with mystery and awe, the promise of magical secrets and ancient knowledge. The soft rhythms of prayers thousands of years old reverberated in my ears and connected me with a tradition whose beginnings lay at the birth of civilization itself. I could sense the deep roots of the past, even if I was not yet able to comprehend them, and they filled me with excitement.

I bounced up the brick stairs to our apartment and leaned on the buzzer eager to report on my new adventure. My father, meanwhile, was lying in wait by the door, just as eager to know what was passing for religious education in the early 1950s. His wide smile and sparkling blue eyes were an invitation to share my excitement. "What did you learn in Sunday school?" he asked. I can remember his deep, loving voice thirty-five years later, as if it were just yesterday.

Climbing into his lap, I showed him the Hebrew alphabet book and the picture book about the prophets that I had just acquired. One illustration showed Moses ascending Mount Sinai to get the Ten Commandments and a bearded, white-haired God peering out from behind the clouds. Daddy began to laugh uproariously, "Do you think God really looks like that, Joanie? Do you think that he lives up there in the clouds?"

I really perked up at his question, because it was something I thought about a lot alone in my room at night, the room with the big windows where the moonlight used to beckon me to think about the heavens. My brother Alan, ten years older, had explained to me that the universe was infinite. I would lie there and try to imagine how big infinity was and how the stars whose expanse was beyond comprehension could have arisen from nothing. I wondered how God Himself had come to be and what the raw materials of creation were. But I always got stuck at the same point: How could God have arisen from nothing? So I deduced that God must always have existed, but this offended my ideas about time, and at about that point I would usually fall asleep. So my father's assertions about where God was and what He looked like were of more than passing Sunday school interest.

I leaned toward him expectantly. "Joanie," he appealed to my seven-year-old intellect, "if God were really a little old man who lived up in the clouds, then airplanes could zoom through his belly button, just like this—right?" He zapped his finger through the air in a convincing demonstration, producing an amazingly resonant airplane sound by forcing a vibrating stream of air through the right side of his mouth.

I giggled at his demonstration, amused but perplexed and disappointed. I wanted answers. "Then where is God?" I demanded. And, with a silent smile, he placed his index finger tenderly on my heart.

LOOKING WITHIN

My father taught me many things, not the least of which was how to win at hide-and-seek. While my friends always sought the deep recesses of closets, bath tubs, and toy chests, I looked for the most obvious places to hide because usually no one thought to check there. There's an old saying, "As above, so below." The same basic strategies and patterns exist at every level of creation, from the orbit of electrons to the movement of the stars. In an old Sufi story, God completed Her handiwork—having created the "many mansions" that the Bible speaks of—the theaters in which the endless variations of the hero's journey back to the Source are played out. Then She looked around for some place to hide while awaiting the return of the souls She had created, their lessons learned and their wisdom won. God chose a place so obvious that we wouldn't think of looking there, for She hid within our hearts.

The connection between the human heart and the Divine Spirit is an ancient archetype that turns up again and again, sometimes in the most unexpected places. I was once giving a seminar on mind/body skills to a group of psychotherapists and physicians in Maine. At the end of the day, a psychiatrist about ten years my senior asked if I had time to talk. Something in her eyes sparked an instant connection between us. We decided to go for a walk in the late afternoon sun of the early fall and were soon enjoying the view from a sleepy country road overlooking the sea. The salt air was fresh, and an eagle soared out over the water, sallying forth from its nest on the craggy cliffs. I breathed in the magnificence and let myself flow back into it. "Sacred time," I thought, because the world seemed to stand still, nature a silent witness to eternity.

Bea was a quiet woman, conservatively dressed, with a slightly professorial air. After we'd walked in silence for several minutes, she turned to me with a look of quiet sincerity. "Something you said today was the final piece of a puzzle that's been falling together for three years. I'd like to tell you the story."

So we sat ourselves down on a fallen log, still warm with September sun, and Bea picked a stalk of grass, heavy with seed. Stroking the fuzzy kernels, she began to scatter them to the wind as she recounted the deep wound of her husband's death. It had been a terrible time for Bea when her husband of twenty years died suddenly from a heart attack. She had felt shattered, bereft, and alone, agonizing about the unfairness of life. At the height of her misery, she dragged herself to a psychiatric conference in Arizona. At the end of her stay, she took a side trip to Sedona, a little town amidst the many-hued buttes sacred to the Navajo Indians. There she came upon a small chapel built into the side of a mountain.

"The chapel was so peaceful, Joan, and so simple. It seemed a natural part of that powerful, sculpted landscape. Looking out, the clouds seemed close enough to touch, and the sky was shimmering, a vibrant blue alive with sunlight. And it was quiet. So quiet. . . . I must have sat there for an hour or so with hardly a thought. It seemed that everything was all right with the world there. It just wasn't possible to worry. The sadness and regrets melted away. What a relief from all the suffering after Sid's death," she sighed.

"After I left the chapel, the peacefulness continued all the way back to my hotel room. I got back about an hour before dinner and lay down to take a nap. No sooner had I closed my eyes than I had a startling lifelike vision. It was like a biblical figure, a female in Mediterranean dress, and she was standing by the bed, no more than three feet from me." Bea paused, drawn by my startled look,

"I know it sounds crazy, Joan, but I actually believe it might have been Mary, the mother of Jesus." She giggled a bit uncomfortably. "Rather unusual for a nice Jewish girl, I suppose. In fact, my next thought was that I had cracked from all the stress and was hallucinating, that I'd become psychotic. I sat up suddenly and snapped open my eyes, but the figure remained. Strangely, I wasn't frightened at all. Just curious."

I was fascinated. "Did she talk to you or communicate in any way?"

Bea nodded, "Yes, but without words. She was smiling at me, gently and lovingly. Her right arm was extended, and she was pointing to my heart. I felt comforted and confused all at once. I knew somehow that this was a message that everything would be—already was—okay. But it also seemed that her gesture was an instruction of some sort. And it was just today, during the workshop when we were discussing the Self, that I realized what the instruction was. She was telling me to look inside, that the answer—the meaning—was there in my own heart." Bea was smiling and crying all at once, and I reached out to touch her shoulder.

"The whole vision lasted for maybe five minutes, but it's been with me every day since, an inspiration and a comfort. But you know, I've only told one other person about it. I mean most people would think I was crazy; even I thought I was crazy at first. As a psychiatrist I'm trained to believe that visions are manifestations of temporal lobe epilepsy or psychosis. There's no framework for explaining them in a positive way. I mean, religious visions? Come on, really. Magical thinking at best." Bea sighed and smiled at me. I could identify with how hard it was for her to talk about something spiritual with an academician. With anybody! Mystical experience is not common parlor conversation.

Bea went on to tell me that she hadn't been to temple since high school because she'd never made a heart connection with her religion. It seemed more like a litany of rules and regulations suited for a culture several thousands of years removed. But, after the vision, she began visiting different temples and churches and had finally found a temple where, much to her surprise, the rabbi talked of worship as a living relationship to God, a mystical experience rather than an academic exercise. Bea discovered Kabbalah, the ancient Jewish mystical tradition, and was surprised to find that its major tenets are similar to Buddhism and, of course, to Christianity, since Jesus's teachings were rooted in the pharisaic Judaism that he preached so eloquently.

I sympathized with Bea's search for a way to really worship. Our family had scoured synagogues, churches, and ashrams in our own search for a form where the Spirit was present. I'll never forget the day that I took our children to attend a church in our new neighborhood after a move. Andrei, then ten, summed it up with the innocence of the Natural Child. "The minister was nice and the food was great. The only trouble is that God wasn't in there." Some of us have been fortunate enough to find the living Spirit in our churches, ashrams, and temples. Others of us find it in nature or in the eyes of a loved one. But God is always present in the heart. She has never forsaken us. Not for an instant. My father's message was the same as Bea's vision: Look within. Seek the place where the Spirit is in hiding, cloaked in the love that is its substance and its action.

A NATION OF CLOSET MYSTICS

Bea's experience is more common than you might think. While many Americans have become disenfranchised from organized religion because it so often fails to meet their spiritual needs, there has been a remarkable increase in direct experiences of the Divine—what are called mystical experiences. In fact, research indicates that a wide variety of seemingly miraculous events—things that we might previously have thought of as supernatural—are getting so commonplace that they seem more and more natural. Since 1973, Andrew Greeley, priest, professor of sociology, and popular author, has been studying Americans' spiritual experiences with his colleagues at the University of Chicago's National Opinions Research Council.

The surveys that Greeley and his colleagues did in 1973 and then repeated in the mid-1980s show that the incidence and variety of "paranormal" experiences ranging from deja vu to contact with the dead have risen sharply. For example, in the 1980s nearly one third of us reported having visions, up from 8 percent in 1973. Half of American adults now believe they have been in contact with a dead loved one, up from about a quarter of the population in 1973. Two thirds of adults report having experienced ESP, up from 58 percent in the earlier survey. One of the questions posed to this random sample of Americans was, Have you ever had a mystical experience, feeling "very close to a powerful, spiritual force that seemed to lift you out of yourself?" An amazing 35 percent of people had, and one seventh of those—5 percent of the population—had literally been "bathed in light" like the apostle Paul.

When pollsters went back to some of these people to get further details, most of them said—as Bea had of her biblical vision—that they had rarely or never shared their experience with another person. Fear of disbelief and ridicule, and, in fundamentalist circles, fear of being denounced as a channel for the "devil" all conspire to keep people in the closet about their mystical experiences. For scientists like me, the problem of ridicule from colleagues is a very real one. No wonder so many of us keep our experiences to ourselves. Daniel Goleman served on an advisory panel for the Institute of Noetic Sciences, founded by former astronaut Edgar Mitchell to explore nonintellectual ways of "knowing." Goleman says:

> Through studies of meditative and other altered states we are beginning to appreciate that alternate modes of knowing can yield truths and understandings that are unavailable to those of us stuck in the mundane reality of everyday consciousness. And the truths understood by mystics may be, from their own vantage point, quite as compelling as those of Western science. . . . I think the evidence is in: we're a nation of closet mystics. And I think the time has arrived when we should come out of the closet.
>
> —*Noetic Sciences Review*, Spring 1987 [p. 7]

There is a common tendency to think that people who have had mystical experiences are either religious fanatics or candidates for locked wards. Greeley's data show exactly the opposite. Those who have had mystical experiences tend to be quite ordinary people, slightly above the median in education and intelligence and a bit below average in their religious involvement. In short, a lot like Bea. When Greeley administered psychological tests to some of these people, such as the ones who had been bathed in light, they scored at the top of the scale for healthy personalities.

A recent Gallup poll confirms Greeley's 1984 data, showing that "paranormal" experiences in the United States are on the rise. An astonishing 5 percent of the population reported in 1981 that they have had a near-death experience, a phenomenon that is often life-changing. Even more amazing to me personally was that 95 percent of Americans reported believing in God or a Universal Spirit. When I saw these data, I joked that the other 5 percent must have all lived in Boston! But as I have gotten braver in asking people about their spiritual outlook, I have indeed found that most people do believe, particularly when the word *God* is substituted for by "Higher Power" or "Universal Spirit," phrases that sidestep early religious experiences that may have felt incomplete or, worse still, damaging.

RELIGION OR SPIRITUALITY?

The increase in mystical experience over the past decade has not been paralleled by an increase in religious involvement. In fact, more of us are avoiding organized religions. A recent Gallup poll found that 78 million Americans either didn't belong to a church or a temple or attended only on infrequent special occasions. That figure is up from 61 million in 1978. Even regular churchgoers had a few bones to pick. The majority felt that churches spent too much time on organizational issues like raising money, and a third considered organized religion too restrictive in its moral teachings. Almost one in four of those polled have turned away from organized religion in search of "deeper spiritual meaning."

Walter Houston Clark, a retired professor of religion from the Andover-Newton Theological Seminary near Boston, spent years researching and writing about the psychology of religion. He started to have profound mystical experiences after many years of teaching academic religion. He likened experiences in the mainstream churches to vaccination. "One goes to church and gets a little something that then protects him or her against the real thing." The often unfulfilling experience of going to church on Sundays or Temple on Saturdays, listening to sermons and saying prayers by rote, led many of us to abandon this concept of religion when it began to feel empty.

Clark's distinction between academic religion and spiritual experience is part of a common thread of wisdom that occurs in all the world's great religions, despite their very real differences. Writer and scientist Aldous Huxley called this thread, which can be traced back for twenty-five centuries, the perennial philosophy.

> In Vedanta and Hebrew Prophecy, in the Tao Teh King and the Platonic dialogues, in the Gospel according to St. John and Mahayana theology, in Plotinus and the Areopagite, among the Persian Sufis and the Christian mystics of the Middle Ages and the Renaissance—the Perennial Philosophy has spoken almost all the languages of Asia and Europe and has made use of the terminology and traditions of every one of the higher religions. . . . The second doctrine of the Perennial Philosophy—that it is possible to know the Divine Ground by a direct intuition higher than discursive reasoning—is to be found in all the great religions of the world. A philosopher who is content merely to know about the ultimate Reality—theoretically and by hearsay—is compared by Buddha to a herdsman of other men's cows . . . (and by Mohammed to) an ass bearing a load of books.
>
> —Aldous Huxley, from his introduction to *The Song of God: Bhagavad-Gita,* translated by Swami Prabhavananda and Christopher Isherwood [pp. 11–12, 15]

Religious upbringing that focuses on learning dogma rather than fostering spiritual experience is not necessarily psychospiritually damaging. It is merely incomplete and may leave us with a sense that our religious tradition is empty. For example, I spent eight summers at a wonderful Jewish camp after my first terrible experience at the "concentration camp" that I described in Chapter Three. Every Friday night we ushered in the Sabbath in the form of a queen surrounded by her attendants. These girls, from different bunks each week, carried candles in the dusk as we sang a beautiful song that I find centering and reconnecting even to this day:

Come O Sabbath Day and bring
Peace and healing on thy wing,
And to every troubled breast,
Speak of thy Divine behest,
Thou shalt rest,
Thou shalt rest.

As we sang, everything would slip away into the peaceful fragrance of the pinegrove where our little service took place. Saturday morning services, in which each bunk likewise participated, and the Saturday evening Havdalah when the Sabbath was ushered out gave a sacred rhythm to the week. But away from camp this sweet experience of ritual and participation was lacking. Temple was for the "high" holy days that seemed more like a fashion show than a time of connection to God. Men mumbled long Hebrew prayers that were incomprehensible, and women were not part of the service.

Missing the sweetness of the pinegrove and the participatory ritual that had created a strong experience of the Self, I began to search for it elsewhere. It was absent in many mainstream churches and temples, unless fellowship, song, and love were an important part of the experience. It tended to be present more frequently wherever the mystical aspects of the world's religions were celebrated. I found it in Christian mysticism, Tibetan Buddhism, Sufism with its ecstatic dances and chants, Hindu Vedanta, and finally, as I came full circle, in Kabbalah, the mystical branch of Judaism.

Unlike mainstream religion, which often reacts with fear or condescension to other religions, mysticism transcends boundaries of all kinds. It is universal and compassionate, and relates to the unities in the great religious traditions rather than to their differences. In all mystical traditions, God is seen as an Inner Divinity as well as a Transcendent Force. In our attempts to find a living connection to God in churches, temples, and ashrams, my husband, Myrin, and I have met a large number of people from a diversity of religious backgrounds who share a common, perennial spiritual vision—the search for the Self. As a society, we are at a time of change in our religious institutions. The old forms have lost some of their life, but new forms have yet to appear. It's a time of spiritual ReVision that challenges us to find the Self within our religious systems, to connect to the powerful rituals that have been alive for millennia, to reclaim the vitality that dogma has too often choked from the system.

RELIGIOUS GUILT

Religion alienates people when it becomes a divisive force rather than a unifying one, when it isolates rather than heals. The most obvious example of diviseness is the strange concept of "holy war," in which the sanctity of human life is violated by killing done in the name of "God." Is God choosing up sides in Ireland, where the Protestants and Catholics are fighting it out, "Christian" against "Christian"? Many people have left religion behind because of this kind of obvious hypocrisy. Others have left it behind because it was psychologically damaging and sometimes a terrible source of guilt. In my practice, I have been shocked at how many people have had early traumatic religious experiences that set them up for a lifetime of religious guilt that is often an unexplored factor in physical disease and mental illness.

Peter, a forty-five-year-old patient who came to see me with recurrent herpes lesions on the buttocks, told me a very sad story about his critical, abusive parents. Both Catholic, his parents had a tremendous fear of Divine retribution. They frightened Peter with talk of mortal sin, a guaranteed ticket to hell. The week's venial sins were listed at the dinner table as well as in the confessional.

Peter grew up terrified of his father, who didn't "spare the rod" to ensure his son's morality. When he finally made his first confession before First Communion, Peter was a nervous wreck. He knew in his heart that he had "coveted Johnny's truck," disobeyed his parents, and, in fact, thought the kind of angry, murderous thoughts about his father that abused children quite normally have. For weeks, Peter agonized about what to tell the priest. And like any small child, he had trouble telling one authority figure from another. Father, priest, and God all seemed like angry parents who would surely find him out and punish him, perhaps mortally.

The priest turned out to be as hardline as Peter's father, handing out long penances over tiny infractions, and he was not a person with whom a small child felt comfortable. Peter also knew he would have to confess all his sins to his parents, since each family member's penance was the usual full disclosure at dinner time. His father added his own brand of penance to that prescribed by the priest, often beating Peter on his buttocks with a belt until red welts appeared. Feeling totally hopeless and scared, Peter soon began to lie. He'd figure the odds: You had to confess *something* or you'd look too good; on the other hand, you had to be careful not to sin too badly. This went on for years, with bitterness and cynicism seeming to replace the fear as Peter grew older.

At forty-five, Peter didn't have much use for his father or the church, but the frightened feelings from childhood had only been repressed, not resolved. When Peter caught herpes as the result of an extramarital affair, his reasonable healthy guilt was overshadowed by unreasonable religious guilt. Even though Peter had long since declared himself an atheist, he soon found that he wasn't. His image of an angry, punitive God had been tucked away, not disposed of; and now he was sure that the herpes was a punishment for his sins. And his body produced an amazing demonstration—breaking out in herpes lesions that mimicked the pattern of his original beatings, a recall of the original psychospiritual trauma.

In Peter's case, mind/body therapy would have been insufficient to deal with the root cause of his illness. He needed both psychotherapy and spiritual redirection to explore and correct the strong religious guilt that had been repressed for so many years. I referred Peter to a pastoral counselor who could serve as a psychospiritual guide in correcting two cases of mistaken identity: Peter's identification of himself as a hopeless sinner, and his identification of God as an unforgiving, punitive destroyer.

Peter's story is not unusual. People often recount similar stories at my workshops on guilt. A woman in Colorado came up to me with tears in her eyes and gave me a long hug, thanking me for confirming what she always knew in her heart—that human beings were intrinsically good. She told me that she had been punished by the nuns in her parochial school when, as an adolescent, she refused to subscribe to the notion of humankind as sinners damaged in the original fall from grace. Believing that her attitude was "dangerous" and would lead her to sin, the nuns apparently felt justified in hitting her.

In the mid-1980s, newspapers carried the particularly shocking account of a little girl who was actually beaten to death by parents who belonged to a fundamentalist Christian cult. One day the child apparently talked back to her parents. In a misguided attempt to save her soul from sin, they spanked her so hard that the blood vessels in her buttocks ruptured and she died from internal bleeding.

Physical abuse in the name of "God" is the most striking way that children come to fear a punitive God, but it is certainly not the only way. Rigid teachings about heaven and hell and about the "saved" and the "unsaved" are similarly damaging. Any religious teaching that pronounces itself to be the only way creates an "us and them" mentality that gives rise to fearful, exclusionary thinking. I will never forget my surprise as a five-year-old when our new housekeeper, a Canadian woman who had been raised in a large, Catholic farm family, washed my hair for the first time. Rubbing my scalp in some disbelief, her eyes grew wide. "My goodness," she said, "Jews don't have horns after all!" When I asked her why she thought we had horns, she told me that her parents had always said so. Jews, after all, were devils. This type of religious training promotes separation between human beings rather than understanding, union, and love. It is certainly not based on scripture, since "love God first and love thy neighbor as thyself" is Jesus's summary of his teachings. Religion is too often twisted to serve as a justification for oppression rather than a system of learning to love.

Religious guilt is the most extreme form of unhealthy guilt because it threatens us with an eternal separation from our Source. Religious guilt also separates us from other people who may have different belief systems. And inevitably religious guilt separates us from ourselves. The healing of this separation comes through "at-one-ment," or atonement, a process of rethinking religious beliefs that may have been spiritually damaging. Reviewing religious beliefs to determine whether they have been spiritually nourishing or spiritually abusive, and then beginning the quest for a spiritually optimistic philosophic or religious outlook is what I call spiritual reVision.

SPIRITUAL REVISION*

The stories of people's spiritual reVisions are always fascinating, and their initiation experiences, at least the ones I've been privileged to hear, fall into three broad categories. First, like Bea, there may be a sudden vision or revelation that descends as an act of grace and completely changes one's spiritual outlook. These grace experiences may follow a period of intense psychological upset or a severe physical trauma culminating in a near-death experience. Second, an accident or physical illness that reminds us of our mortality often spurs a spiritual search, because, as priorities fall suddenly into place, questions about life's meaning also tend to arise. Third, the realization that addictions stem from identification with a false self that lacks either the wisdom or the strength to overcome its fearful behaviors has led many people to spiritual reVision as part of healing addiction.

Through the years, I've been privileged to hear many people's transformation experiences. Just hearing these stories often has a profound effect on the listeners. The most informative lecture about the Self lacks the impact of a single personal account, so at workshops I often ask people to share "holy moments," dreams, images, visions, or near-death experiences.

Marcie, a thirty-five-year-old software engineer, almost died in the hospital from a severe allergic reaction to penicillin in her late twenties. Prior to her experience, she knew nothing of the "core" out-of-body events that have been so well described by near-death researchers such as Drs. Raymond Moody and Kenneth Ring (you can find references to their books in Chapter Ten) and that have since been widely publicized. Marcie told a group of us how incredible it was to read accounts of other people's near-death experiences more than a year after her own, and to see that, although each one was as different as a fingerprint, they were all basically alike. Each experience had key similarities—leaving the body, speeding down a tunnel, emerging into a loving light, reviewing one's life, and finally returning to the body. Of course, not every person experiences all the elements Marcie had. I hope that I can do justice to the magnificence of her story in the retelling.

Marcie took a deep breath and settled into her chair, her eyes focused inwardly, as she began to recall the experience of her near death. In a

*A term borrowed from the journal *ReVision: The Journal of Consciousness and Change*, Heldref Publications, Washington, D.C.

soft, clear voice, she told us that "I—that is the intelligence that I identify as me—floated free from my body. I saw it lying there in the bed, more of a curiosity than anything else—like the clothes you step out of before going to bed at night. You use them, but they aren't you. Then, in a flash, I felt myself propelled down a tunnel toward an incredibly warm, indescribably brilliant light. It was exactly like descriptions I've read since, but no description can possibly do it justice. All I can say is that the light is totally loving and safe. You want to cry tears of joy, being in it. It is really like a homecoming. You are so grateful to be back in that familiar state. The light is all around you and seems also to come from inside you. You are the light and it is you, and it is connected at once to everything else in the universe. The light is conscious and intelligent, and in it you share that intelligence. Suddenly everything that has happened in your life makes complete sense." She shook her head, still amazed by the experience.

"The whole meaning and purpose of life was clear. I could see that the events in my life had each happened for a reason, and that the reason had to do with building enough faith to recognize that love is the force that holds the universe together. The only lesson we're here to learn is the lesson of love. Suddenly the worn-out phrase that God is Love was totally clear. It's the truth. It really is." She looked up and glanced around the room at each of us.

Everyone's attention was riveted on Marcie, and many people were in tears. She continued on, her face and voice soft with the love of which she spoke. "I realized some very personal things about what I was learning through my life. Then I knew that I had to return to my body to carry on with these learnings. Since that time, I have lost my fear of death. I just don't believe in it anymore."

Once we have had a mystical experience like Marcie or Bea, it calls up our previous beliefs for questioning, replacing *concepts* about God with an actual *experience* of God. Mystics have written about their experiences of the Divine for centuries, usually summarizing them as "ineffable"—beyond words. Nonetheless, the words that people do use to explain these encounters with the Divine have a commonality. They often pertain to the very real and brilliant experience of light and a feeling of overpowering love and opening of the heart that are typical of near-death experiences. As Andrew Greeley's poll showed, they are also common to the transcendent mystical experiences that another 5 percent of the American public has reported.

David was a man in his early sixties who came to the Mind/Body Clinic with severe arthritis in his hips and knees. He was in terrible pain most of the time, despite a regimen of aspirin and treatments with gold. He had just taken an early retirement from his successful printing business. Feeling out of control and depressed, David had decided to try meditation and imagery to put himself back in the driver's seat. About eight weeks into the program, he called me aside from the group and asked for an individual appointment. He was very excited and wanted to explain how and why his pain had suddenly vanished a few weeks before.

When the day finally came for our appointment, David looked at me very sheepishly. "Promise me that you won't think I'm crazy," he said, leaning closer to me, speaking almost in a whisper, as if afraid to be overheard. "It was about four weeks ago. I was asleep in my bed, when suddenly I had the funniest feeling. It was like the air in the room had suddenly become electric. Then I sensed a presence at the bedroom door. I know this sounds like the 'The Twilight Zone,' Joan, but stay with me. I know I'm not imagining this, and I'm sure I haven't gone crazy." David's eyes grew large at the memory as he continued. "I turned around and saw a ball of incredibly bright light hovering in the doorway. It was made out of—I don't know any other way to put this," he said, drawing in a tentative breath and lowering his voice even more, "but—well, love energy."

"Love energy?" I inquired. "What is that like, David, what do you mean?"

"There's no way to explain it really—you just know you're in the presence of God—held and loved. It moved over to the bed and enveloped me. It filled me. It *was* me. That was the most incredible thing: The light outside me seemed to awaken a light inside me, and they were one and the same." He paused reverently at the recollection. "And a moment later it was gone, and so was the pain. I jumped out of bed and started doing knee bends. I was able—there was no pain and no stiffness! And beyond that, Joan, my fear was gone, too. In that moment, I understood that what they call God is actually love and that it's the very electricity that runs the body. Can you imagine that?!"

David paused for a moment and then continued, "Afterward the pain stayed away entirely for about three days, then began to come back, but milder than before. Now when I feel it, I drop quickly into a meditative state by using the diaphragmatic breathing and then I just imagine the light. I inhale the light through the top of my head and let it fill me, part by part, until I am buzzing with the kind of energy that filled the room that night. Then the pain goes away, and I'm left with a feeling of peace and contentment."

The real transformation that such mystical events creates is a spiritual reVision—the conversion of fear and doubt into a trust in God and the workings of the universe. They are a powerful cure for helplessness and pessimism. Furthermore, they are contagious. When one person's belief system and frame of mind changes, that person affects other people positively, just by their presence, even if the others do not share the experience on which the transformation was based. Andrew Greeley comments that:

> A small minority, maybe under 20 million, have undergone profoundly religious moments of ecstasy. They report out of body trips, being bathed in light or other encounters that transform their lives. They become profoundly trusting, convinced that something good rules in the world. Whether their number is growing or they're just now ready to tell about it, that many people capable of trust can have a lasting effect on the country.
>
> —"The 'Impossible': It's Happening,"
> *American Health*, January/February 1987

ENLIGHTENMENT AND THE DARK NIGHT OF THE SOUL

Enlightenment is a shift in identity. Instead of identifying with the temporal, collective false self called the ego, we shift our identity to the eternal Self. While many have glimpses of enlightenment, few of us hold on to the realization of the Self as a permanent state. During her near-death experience, Marcie was in a state of enlightenment. She knew who she really was, what the meaning and purpose of her life were, and she was immersed in a blissful mystical union with the all-loving, all-forgiving mystical splendor of the light. The same was true of David after his encounter with the light. But, returning to everyday life, both of them still found that they had plenty of ego identification left. Having had the grace of an enlightenment experience, they were able to see their false identifications a little bit more easily, but they still had to work through them. Enlightenment was a flash of possibility, a gift of grace that lead to spiritual reVision rather than a permanent state.

The process of working through our false identifications has been compared to peeling off the layers of an onion. You get through one layer and feel a lot better because the inner light and vitality of the Self can shine through more clearly. You get used to functioning with this increased level of energy and insight, and then, sure enough, you bump into another piece of your shadow. You feel temporarily worse again as you go through the process of recognizing and integrating yet another false identity. The deeper into the onion you go, the bigger the shadow dragons you will encounter, because you have the energy and insight to see them, integrate them, and move on once again. During the process of moving deeper into the onion, people often go through a terribly difficult period when they uncover some of their darkest shadow secrets. During this period, it is common to lose one's faith in the Self and in the journey, and to feel desperately afraid and alone.

This difficult period has been called the dark night of the soul. It is the death of a big shadow dragon. Its successful completion leads to a rebirth that brings one much closer to living from the Self or, in some cases, to a permanent state of enlightenment. Such was the case of Rabbi Isaac Eizik of Komarno, a Hasidic master who lived from 1806 to 1874. His secret diary, *Megillat Setarim*, published in the 1940s, deals in part with the death/rebirth experience of his enlightenment. He worked on himself for many years and expended great effort in studying and praying. Then he spoke of going through a time of great spiritual "dryness," when his previous enthusiasm faded away. For months, it was nearly impossible for him to pray or to study, and he finally became quite seriously depressed. A *dark night* came over his soul and:

> . . . much bitterness passed over my head as a result of these blandishments, really more bitter than a thousand times death. But once I had overcome these blandishments, suddenly, in the midst of the day, as I was studying . . . a great light fell upon me. The whole house became filled with light, a marvelous light, the Shekhinah resting there. This was the first time in my life that I had some little taste of His light, may He be blessed. It was authentic without error or confusion, a wondrous delight and a most pleasant illumination beyond all comprehension.
>
> —*Jewish Mystical Testimonies*, edited by Louis Jacobs [pp. 240–41]

The Shekhinah is the divine presence of God in its female aspect, what the Hindus would call Shakti. Its closest approximation in Christian thought is the Holy Spirit, the Comforter. It often comes when the heart has been ripped apart—broken open—by psychic pain, when the psychological defenses that keep us out of touch with the shadow are weakened or rendered useless. When the shadow is seen so clearly, the illusion of the "perfect" false self suddenly breaks down and the mask that we have falsely identified with is shattered. At this point, it's no wonder we experience what the rabbi spoke of as a bitterness more than "a thousand times death," for it is actually the death of our ego. If we succeed in tolerating this bitterness, then the light of the Self will begin to shine more brightly, and the presence of the Comforter will grow stronger. Those few who stay centered in the Self, as did Rabbi Eizik, without reconstructing any new ego filters, become permanently enlightened, or Self-realized.

GRACE

People who have had significant spiritual reVisions, whether through mystical experience, the "sacred wound" of intense psychological pain or illness, or healing addiction all say the same thing. Their change of heart was an experience of grace. In *Minding the Body, Mending the Mind,* I told the story of a young physician named Sam, who had AIDS. The story is so meaningful to me that it occupies the entire final chapter of the book. I'll retell just a small part of it here.

Sam and I originally met when I was called to his hospital room to teach him how to meditate. What began as a professional encounter deepened into an extraordinary friendship through which both of us found a renewal of faith and a spiritual reVision. The grace of our short time together was captured serendipitously in an experience we shared concerning the old spiritual "Amazing Grace." One Sunday morning in the early spring, I set out for the long ride to the hospital where Sam lay dying. The promise of new life had begun to explode in crocuses and fat green buds, and I was in a bittersweet frame of mind. I was sad because of the suffering Sam had endured and because I would miss him, but I felt heartened at what we had learned together. I also felt a sense of celebration that his soul would soon be free, reborn back to the Spirit. A peace settled over me and I found myself singing "Amazing Grace," over and over for most of the hour's drive to the hospital.

When I arrived in Sam's room, he was surrounded by loved ones. I hugged him and then hung around his neck a medallion that was a symbol of soul and Spirit, the intersection of the material and noetic realms. Then we held hands and looked into one another's eyes with all the love we had shared in our year together. Sam smiled and made a surprising request. He asked me to sing "Amazing Grace." Only later that day, when one of his friends played a beautiful rendition by Leontyne Price, did I find out it was one of Sam's favorite songs. That was the last time I saw Sam before he died.

Several days later, Myrin and I were in New Orleans on business. We were sad because Sam's memorial service had been held earlier that day and we had missed being there. As we walked through the French Quarter, talking about Sam and wishing him well, a saxophonist stepped out from a doorway and caught our eye. Nodding his head, he lifted the saxophone to the sky and played "Amazing Grace." You can invoke coincidence if you'd like, but I agree with surgeon and healer Bernie Siegel, M.D., who says, "Coincidence is just God's way of remaining anonymous."

Grace is an ancient theological concept that Webster's dictionary defines in four ways: a) the free and unmerited love and favor of God; b) divine influence acting in man to restrain him from sin; c) a state of reconciliation to God; and d) spiritual instruction, improvement, and edification. But grace is more than a concept. It is a living act and expression of the natural laws by which love extends itself. The impetus to make the hero's journey, to search for the Self, to be reconciled with God, is an act of grace. That's what the old spiritual tells us so well in the musical language of the heart: "Amazing grace, how sweet the sound that saved a soul like me. I once was lost, but now I'm found, was blind but now I see." Grace restores our spiritual vision so that we can see where we're going.

Grace comes unearned and unsought. The Indian sage Ramakrishna taught that the winds of grace are blowing perpetually; we have just to raise our sails. Jesus explained grace by using an "as above, so below" metaphor about loving-kindness. God gives His children what they need, just as earthly parents do. But, in addition to grace as a free, unsought gift, our actions also attract an additional measure. To extend Jesus's metaphor, when our children show an interest in what we're teaching them, we naturally respond by putting a little extra energy into the lessons. This second kind of grace is a little like a universal matching grant that helps us along our way. It is a powerful force—a reality—that works in a reproducible manner.

Several years ago, my dear friend Rachel Naomi Remen, a talented physician and healer, explained this second type of grace to me. We were sitting in a Mexican restaurant in northern California, and I was pouring my heart out about one of my oldest and most resistant false selves, the victim. I had donned the victim mask partially as a result of the humiliation I suffered when I ran away from camp as a seven-year-old and partially because of my relationship with my mother. Courage and power were stuffed into my shadow as a result of my public shaming at the camp and the many more subtle shamings in my home. A victim self was born.

Unable to handle difficult situations by the honest and straightforward expression of needs and feelings, the victim hopes for salvation by engaging the pity of the oppressor. Victims *need* aggressors to oppress them. We can then feel enraged at our ill treatment, which is how we compensate for helplessness and fear, experiencing a temporary surge of power in the adrenaline rush. Like Snow White, I recognized this old ego pattern, but I had been unable to escape it, and I had gotten myself into an angry hole. I was despondent about my ability to change. "After all," I lamented to Rachel, "the conditioning runs too deep. How can you let go of patterns you have been living for a lifetime?" I was disgusted and disheartened.

Rachel leaned toward me at that candlelit table, her eyes and voice filled with love and reassurance. She picked up the butter spreader from her dish and laid it across her finger, inviting me to a new perspective. "Joanie," she said, "picture a seesaw resting on a fulcrum. You work to move the board until—at the 50 percent mark—it teeters on the balance point."

I was transfixed as *I watched* the spreader. "At 51 percent," Rachel continued, "the balance suddenly shifts." The spreader tilted instantly at the tiniest pressure. Rachel smiled. "See? You need to work hard, all right, but the other 49 percent is a gift from God. It is called grace."

At that moment, something really shifted. I had a new vision, a spiritual reVision that gave me hope, and since that day I've seen the wisdom of Rachel's words demonstrated in many lives, time and time again. The day of our talk, I'd estimate that I was about 35 percent of the way toward understanding and moving beyond my childhood victim self. Over the next year or so, when we'd talk on the phone, I'd report on the progress—40 percent, 45 percent. Rachel warned me that the last few percent were always the hardest, since the ego self—the false personality—resents being squeezed out and fights for its life. She was right. But one day, in the midst of the old familiar pattern, I decided I'd had enough and I left a professional relationship in which I had stayed for too long feeling like an angry victim. It wasn't easy, nor was it done with a lot of finesse, but I did it. And it was the 51 percent point, the turning point. Since then, the old pattern has been much easier to spot and avert. But healing from old patterns is not an all-or-nothing matter. We get many opportunities to practice being aware of our conditioned reactions and to make new choices. Sometimes we succeed and sometimes we fail, in spite of our best efforts to change, but grace can certainly tip the odds in our favor.

Grace can be attracted, most simply, by asking for help. This is the perennial psychospiritual wisdom of "knock and it shall be opened." At times when the victim role comes up for me and I feel almost irresistibly pulled back toward that familiar and loathsome pattern of my past, I pray. I let God know that *I am aware* of my predicament and that *I need help*. This admission of personal powerlessness creates a critical shift in attitude. Rather than feeling like a helpless child who is a prisoner of the past, I really feel like a beloved child of God. In the latter role, I can depend on the Divine Spirit to move through me with much greater wisdom, power, and love than my limited ego can provide, freeing me from the need to feel like a victim. When we can use adversity and the continued pull of old patterns to provide the impetus for prayer and the shift to becoming children of God, miracles begin to happen in every area of our lives because we have opened our sails to the winds of grace. And, as the old spiritual says, that grace shall lead us home.

GRACE, LOVE, AND AWARENESS

There are two basic emotions—fear and love. In fear, the ego closes down in self-protection, and our awareness of life constricts to the immediate worry or difficulty on our mind. We can't see any new possibilities. Instead, our mind is all made up about what our experience will be. Both mind and heart are closed like steel traps, and we are caught in our own fear. In love, both heart and mind are open to the myriad possibilities of life. Experiences are new and fresh. We are often delighted and surprised. We literally see more closely into the richness of life. We can appreciate subtle hues and patterns, smell complex fragrances, and feel a depth of feeling that brings us into the fullness of life. This is what Luigi Galvani called the enchantment of the heart.

Driving down the highway, the trees and hills may suddenly come alive, their splendor filling the moment. Or a tree that we have seen many times before suddenly looks entirely different with a thin coat of snow or ice, and we appreciate its beauty afresh. Or we look into the face of a friend or our beloved, and for some reason we stop seeing them as a collection of our own memories and projections, and we see the Self in them. These are holy moments during which we enter into the state of grace that is perpetually available to us.

While grace is always present as an outpouring of Divine love, sometimes our sails are tightly furled and we cannot open to the gift of life. When we're too busy thinking about errands and other commitments to be present to the act of lovemaking, our hearts are closed and we lose out. When worry overtakes the mind, we can't enjoy our food. Have you ever eaten a whole meal and barely tasted a bite because your attention was somewhere else? We can be physically present at the most glorious sunset, but when the mind is wandering, we don't receive the beauty. When our cup is full of fear, preoccupation, or concepts, there is little room for grace. Playwright Eugene Ionesco expressed it this way, in *Present Past, Past Present*:

> Once, long ago, I was sometimes overcome by a sort of grace, a euphoria. It was as if, first of all, every notion, every reality was emptied of its content. After this emptiness . . . , it was as if I found myself suddenly at the center of pure ineffable existence; it was as if things had freed themselves of all arbitrary labels, of a framework that didn't suit them, that limited them; social and logical constraint or the need to define them, to organize them, disappeared.

Thich Nhat Hanh, a Vietnamese Buddhist teacher and poet, presents a practical approach to emptying our cups of concepts and being open to grace using the Buddhist practice of mindfulness, or present-centered awareness. In his beautiful little book *Being Peace*, he says: "Life is filled with suffering, but it is also filled with many wonders, like the blue sky, the sunshine, the eyes of a baby. To suffer is not enough. We must also be in touch with the wonders of life. They are within us and all around us, everywhere, any time" (p. 1). He instructs us in opening the heart:

> I would like to offer one short poem you can recite from time to time, while breathing and smiling.
>
> *Breathing in, I calm body and mind.*
> *Breathing out, I smile.*
> *Dwelling in the present moment*
> *I know this is the only moment.*
>
> *"Breathing in, I calm body and mind."* This line is like drinking a glass of ice water—you feel the cold, the freshness, permeate your

body. When I breathe in and recite this line, I actually feel the breathing calming my body, calming my mind.

"Breathing out, I smile." You know the effect of a smile. A smile can relax hundreds of muscles in your face, and relax your nervous system. That is why the Buddhas and Bodhisattvas are always smiling. When you smile, you realize the wonder of the smile.

"Dwelling in the present moment." While I sit here, I don't think of somewhere else, of the future or of the past. I sit here, and know where I am. This is very important. . . . We tend to postpone being alive to the future, the distant future, we don't know when. . . . Therefore the technique, if we have to speak of a technique, is to be in the present moment, to be aware of the here and now. . . .

"I know this is the only moment." This is the only moment that is real. To be here and now, and enjoy the present moment is our most important task. "Calming, Smiling, Present moment, Only moment." I hope you will try it.

***Stop for a few minutes** and try the techniques expressed in Thich Nhat Hanh's beautiful poem of mindfulness. Be present with each breath, each verse. This is a powerful technique, deceptive in its utter simplicity, and a great help in being present to the gift of grace. Like witnessing, it is a technique of centering. Cutting the cords that bind you to past and future, these two conscious, intentional breaths can restore you to the Self, to Now. Over time, this poem is like a portable Buddhist master. It teaches you to be mindful, nonjudgmentally present and aware of life. Alive again.*

Mindfulness opens the door to joy—and therefore to gratitude. The great Christian mystic Meister Eckhart commented that "if 'thank you' was the only prayer we ever said, it would be enough." "Thank you" completes the circuit between creator and creation. It signifies that we have received the gift that creation is trying to bestow on us, that we have allowed God's love and grace to become manifest. This is a profound understanding of creation that has been explained in many different ways. The philosopher Martin Heidegger put it very simply: "This is man's essential calling—to bring the world into being." We do this by receiving with an open heart. In gratitude, we realize that life, God, and the Self are one, as was said so well by the Russian Orthodox priest St. John of Kronstadt, who lived in the late nineteenth and early twentieth century.

Prayer is a state of continual gratitude.
If I do not feel a sense of joy
in God's creation, if I forget

to offer the world back to God
with thankfulness
I have advanced very little
upon the Way.
I have not yet learnt
to be truly human.
For it is only in thanksgiving
that I can become myself.

SUGGESTIONS FOR THE READER

1. What was your childhood teaching about God? Did it help you to establish a spiritual connection or has it hindered you? You may want to write your memories, thoughts, and feelings in a journal.

2. Practice Thich Nhat Hanh's poem of mindfulness if you find it appealing, or just remember to take a few breaths often during the day, and to return to the witness, to the Now. Let yourself feel the gratitude and contentment that naturally accompany opening your awareness to grace.

CHAPTER SEVEN

From Religious Guilt to Spiritual Optimism

Two young men with AIDS, John and Mark, were patients of mine. Both were furious at the twist of fate that would ultimately take their lives. Both had periods of intense anxiety and depression. But there the similarities ended. John regarded AIDS as the grand finale of a life not worth living and as God's punishment for being gay. Mark viewed AIDS as a difficult passage, but he used the nearness of death as a way to enhance his appreciation of life and his closeness to the Divine.

Being with Mark was like being with a child. In the midst of a serious discussion, his face would often light up with joy as he caught sight of the world outside the window. The antics of a bird, the play of light and shadow in the leaves, were ever-new sources of wonder to him. "Chronicle," a Boston television magazine show, followed Mark around with a camera for the last two years of his life. They documented the full range of his emotional vitality, his joy and delight, as well as the emotions that we often try to deny as "negative." Mark's sadness, his fear, and his voluble rage against society's treatment of gays and other minorities regarded as "different" or "inferior" gave depth and authenticity to his intense engagement with life. Mark didn't fear death; rather, he gave himself to it grudgingly because he cherished life as sacred. Mark ranked medically as a long-term survivor before he died in the fall of 1988.

John, on the other hand, greeted the news of his disease with a resigned, "Well, I figured I'd get AIDS sooner or later." He had never forgiven his parents, a smothering mother and a distant father, for making his life "neurotically miserable." Seeing no further point to life, and tormented by the idea that AIDS was God's punishment for his sins, John immediately left the law firm where he practiced and went into a deep depression. He saw no meaning in life, temporal or eternal. Only two months after his diagnosis, John died from a severe bout with pneumocystis pneumonia.

Viktor Frankl, the noted psychiatrist who survived four Nazi death camps, wrote an eloquent distillation of his experiences in the book *Man's Search for Meaning*. It didn't take the young Frankl long to notice that people who gave up the will to live—who lost faith that there was any meaning in their lives—soon died of the epidemics that ran rampant through the camps. A Dutch Jew named Etty Hillesum, who eventually perished in Auschwitz, noticed much the same thing, which she recorded in her inspiring journals, miraculously recovered and published as *An Interrupted Life: The Diaries of Etty Hillesum, 1941–1943*. Commenting on meaning and survival, she says:

> There is a limit to suffering, perhaps no human being is given more than he can shoulder—beyond a certain point we just die. People are dying here even now of a broken spirit, because they can no longer find any meaning in life, young people. The old ones are rooted in firmer soil and accept their fate with dignity and calm. You see so many different sorts of people here and so many attitudes to the hardest, the ultimate questions [p. 247].

Etty moved through the many camps she lived in, until she was finally gassed in Auschwitz, giving the only thing she had left—and ultimately the thing that matters most: compassion. Etty made the hero's journey into a "land removed from everyday reality" in desperate circumstances, yet she saw her circumstances much as Mark came to see his AIDS. Instead of rejecting either her circumstances or herself as bad or evil as John did, Etty lived life fully in the camps. The following lines from her journal made a lasting impression on me:

> People sometimes say, "You must try to make the best of things." I find this such a feeble thing to say. Everywhere things are both very good and very bad at the same time. The two are in balance, everywhere and always. I never have the feeling that I have got to make the best of things, everything *is* fine just as it is. Every situation, however miserable, is complete in itself and contains the good as well as the bad [p. 254].

As I read that statement by Etty, the perennial wisdom of taking the "middle way" between the pairs of opposites—good and evil, light and dark, mask and shadow—came to life for me. Etty's ability to live life with passion and compassion, despite being surrounded by the horrors of a concentration camp, is a real-life demonstration of finding the mythological Grail. The middle way is path of wisdom that informs the decision about when to fight for change and when to accept our circumstances. The middle way walked by contemporary heros such as Etty is the same path of which the Buddha and Jesus spoke. The ancients told us that it was as "narrow as the razor's edge."

WHY DO BAD THINGS HAPPEN?

When something bad happens, our basic survival instincts are triggered, and we try to get back in control by figuring out *why* it happened so that we can prevent its recurrence. Otherwise we remain in the vulnerable state of helplessness that follows sudden shocks to our worldview.

The state of helplessness has been the subject of wide-ranging psychological and physiological research, as I discuss at length in *Minding the Body, Mending the Mind*. Psychologically, helplessness sets the stage for anxiety, depression, pessimism, and guilty thinking. Physiologically, helplessness can provoke sudden cardiac death, as discussed by University of Pennsylvania psychologist Martin Seligman in his fine book *Helplessness: On Depression, Development and Death*; or it can lead to chronic immune suppression, as Seligman and his colleagues have shown more recently. They have also demonstrated that rodents made helpless experimentally by their inability to control the "bad events" of intermittent shocks are significantly less able to reject cancer cells than mice who received the same amount of shock but had the opportunity to turn it off.

Understanding what we think about life's bad events gives us valuable information about where we are psychologically on the continuum between helplessness and the control that Etty demonstrated, a control grounded in compassion and self-knowledge. Our ideas about why bad things happen also reflect our religious beliefs and spiritual focus, as we saw in the cases of Mark and John. Psychology and religion are two sides of the same coin. They meet in our ideas about what creates the events of our lives. There are three basic ways that we think about the genesis of bad events. We can attribute problems to ourselves, to some person or force outside of ourselves, or to chance.

If we look to ourselves as the cause of our troubles, we can either take responsibility for our actions in a way that leads to insight and growth, or we can engage in self-blame. Seligman found that chronic self-blamers are pessimists who explain life's troubles with a triad of internal, global, and stable attributions. Take as an example a young student who fails an algebra exam. Internal explanations point the finger of blame at oneself (for instance, "I'm stupid or lazy") rather than at something external, such as bad teaching. Global means that I'm stupid in general rather than in algebra alone ("I'm gonna flunk English and Spanish, too, because I'm a poor student"). Stable means the problem is going to last forever. Our pessimistic student might comment that "I'll never be any good at learning," rather than invoke a temporary explanation like "this semester's courses are particularly difficult" or "my reading problem can be mastered." Pessimism reflects underlying helplessness and leads to depression rather than to responsible action.

If we attribute our problems to others, we can do it in four basic ways. We can blame other people or society at large, disowning our own responsibility and foregoing the insights we might have gleaned from the event. We can also attribute our problems to a powerful force, such as fate, which likewise results in disowning responsibility. The third attribution we can make involves God. God's intervention can be viewed as benevolent (an act of His will that we may not understand but still believe is for our good) or malevolent (God is punishing us for our sins). The fourth external attribution we can make is to Satan: "The devil made me do it," or the devil caused this to happen. Projecting our own or society's collective shadow onto a psychic bogeyman likewise blocks responsibility and growth.

If we attribute our problems to chance, we sidestep the issues of blame and responsibility, and the perennial question of why a loving God would allow humankind to suffer. When Rabbi Harold Kushner's beloved son died of the rare disease of rapid aging called progeria, the rabbi neither blamed himself for his son's illness, nor did he blame God. In his book *When Bad Things Happen to Good People*, he invoked chance, reasoning that the universe is still incompletely formed and that within the part where chaos still reigns, bad events can happen, even though God is loving. While this attribution spares us guilt feelings, it doesn't make us feel any less helpless. In fact, it makes us feel even more helpless because there is no way to control, manipulate, bargain with, avoid, or pray to chance. Dr. Elaine Pagels, Professor of Religion at Princeton University, asserts that human beings have traditionally preferred to invoke guilt and Divine punishment as an explanation for why bad things happen, precisely in order to avoid feelings of helplessness.

The guiltier and more helpless we feel, the more we want a black-and-white answer for why bad things happen. In my own experience, an insistence on knowing *why* can sometimes prevent us from keeping an open heart and mind in coping with the situation, whatever its cause. Yet taking responsibility for meeting life's difficulties with awareness and courage does involve an exploration of why bad things happen. Consider this scenario. George is fifty-six years old and develops lung cancer. He has been a heavy smoker all his life. There is a physical why here—the cigarettes. However, data show that single, widowed, and divorced men are likelier to die from cigarette-related causes than married men. George has been divorced for seven years, so perhaps there is also a psychological why. The next level of question would be whether there was a spiritual why. For some people, this inquiry might take the form, "Is God punishing George?" or, for others, "Is George's cancer karmic, the result of past actions?" As we will see, both these viewpoints can become limiting and guilt inducing.

The only "spiritual data" I can refer to as a scientist are reports of people who have had near-death experiences and the very small data base on reincarnation. None of these sources implies that bad events like George's lung cancer are punishments. What they do imply is that our own limited perception of the different levels of consciousness is too narrow for most of us to understand spiritual "reasons." Consider the experience of psychiatrist Brian Weiss, as reported in his book *Many Lives, Many Masters*. When he hypnotized his patient Catherine, she began to relive a series of what Weiss accepts as past lives. In the interval between lives, she could serve as a channel for what Weiss called the Masters, as well as a conduit for information about Weiss's father and infant son, who were both dead. Weiss says:

> The greatest tragedy in my life had been the unexpected death of our first born son, Adam, who was only twenty-three days old when he died, early in 1971. About ten days after we had brought him home from the hospital he had developed respiratory problems and projectile vomiting. The diagnosis was extremely difficult to make. "Total anomalous pulmonary veinous drainage with an atrial septal defect," we were told. "It occurs once in approximately every ten million births." The pulmonary veins, which were supposed to bring oxygenated blood back to the heart, were incorrectly routed, entering the heart from

> the wrong side. It was as if his heart were turned around, *backward*. Extremely, extremely rare [p. 55].

Weiss was caught completely by surprise when Catherine, who knew nothing at all about his family, told him the following during the state she entered between recollection of her own lifetimes.

> Your father is here, and your son, who is a small child. Your father says you will know him because his name is Avrom, and your daughter is named after him. Also, his death was due to his heart. Your son's heart was also important, for it was backward, like a chicken's. He made a great sacrifice for you out of his love. His soul is very advanced.

Catherine went on to explain that Adam had taken birth for the sake of his parents. The Buddhists call this kind of soul a *bodhisattva*—one who takes on a body for the benefit of others rather than for their own soul growth, which has already progressed past the need for physical incarnation. Weiss's experience puts a very different slant on the age-old question, "How can God let little babies die?"

GUILT: THE INTERFACE BETWEEN PSYCHOLOGY AND RELIGION

> Now the serpent was more subtle than any other wild creature that the Lord God had made. He said to the woman, "Did God say, 'You shall not eat of any tree of the garden'?" And the woman said to the serpent, "We may eat of the fruit of the trees of the garden; but God said, 'You shall not eat of the fruit of the tree which is in the midst of the garden, neither shall you touch it, lest you die.' " But the serpent said to the woman, "You will not die. For God knows that when you eat of it your eyes will be opened, and you will be like God, knowing good and evil." So when the woman saw that the tree was good for food, and that it was a delight to the eyes, and that the tree was desired to make one wise, she took of its fruit and ate; and she also gave some to her husband, and he ate. Then the eyes of both were opened, and they knew that they were naked; and they sewed fig leaves together and made themselves aprons.
>
> —*The Book of Genesis* 3:1–8, Revised Standard Edition

The third chapter of Genesis continues as Adam and Eve, with their new power of discrimination, feel shame at their nakedness and hide from God, who is walking in the garden. When God sees their shame, He knows that they have disobeyed Him and eaten of the tree of knowledge of good and evil. He punishes the serpent by condemning it to crawl on its belly for the rest of its days and creating enmity between its offspring and Eve's. He punishes Eve, and womankind, by multiplying pain in childbearing and subjugating women to men. He punishes Adam, and mankind, by making him toil in the fields for a living until death. Then God drives the couple out of Eden and posts the cherubim, with a flaming sword, to guard the way to the tree of life, lest Adam who "has become like one of us, knowing good and evil" should eat of the tree and become immortal like the gods.

In her scholarly yet readable book *Adam, Eve and the Serpent*, Elaine Pagels traces the history of how this story has shaped Western culture. Whereas early Christians believed that humankind was blessed by God in the gifts of nature and in the moral freedom that allowed Eve to exercise free will in the garden, in the late fourth and early fifth century St. Augustine reinterpreted the story and introduced what Pagels calls

> . . . a doctrine that categorically denied the goodness of creation and the freedom of the will. . . . Augustine emphasizes humanity's enslavement to sin. Humanity is sick, suffering, and helpless, irreparably damaged by the fall, for that "original sin," Augustine insists, involved nothing else than Adam's prideful attempt to establish his own autonomous self-government [p. 99].

How did Augustine come to believe that all mankind was tainted by sin as a result of Adam and Eve's disobedience in the garden and their subsequent "fall" from grace? Both Pagels and the highly outspoken Dominican Catholic priest Matthew Fox cite Augustine's battle with his sexual impulses, which he discusses in his *Confessions*. Augustine chronicled his natural, adolescent sexual urges and the humiliation of discovering that the sexual organ has a will of its own and doesn't necessarily obey one's bidding. From this, Augustine rashly concluded that the whole concept of free will was only an illusion. Pagels quotes Augustine's conclusion about why he suffered from enslavement by impulses that were beyond his will: "I was not, therefore, the cause of it, but the sin that dwells in me: from the punishment of that more voluntary sin, because I was a son of Adam" (p. 107).

Augustine, you may appreciate from our previous discussion, managed to sidestep his feelings of helplessness by blaming the sexuality he wished to repress on someone else—in this case, on Adam, who was tempted by Eve, who in turn was tempted by the serpent. Augustine chose the impersonal guilt of original sin rather than admit personal helplessness over natural impulses that had grown larger than life, as impulses will, when we label them as evil and stuff them into the long bag of the shadow.

While Augustine's personal commitment to the doctrine of original sin is understandable, Pagels pondered the question of why Christians in general would have subscribed to his notion, antithetical as it was to the prevalent beliefs in the goodness of man. She directs our attention once more to the instinctual questions that arise from human suffering, "Why has this happened, and why has this happened to me?" She concludes that:

> Augustine's answer simultaneously acknowledges and denies human helplessness; in this paradox, I suspect, its power lies. To the sufferer, Augustine says, in effect, "You *personally* are not to blame for what has come upon you; the blame goes back to our father, Adam, and our mother, Eve." Augustine assures the sufferer that pain is unnatural, death an enemy, alien intruders upon normal human existence, and thus he addresses the deep human longing to be free of pain. But he also assures us that suffering is neither without meaning nor without specific cause. Both the cause and the meaning of suffering, as he sees it, lie in the sphere of *moral choice*, not *nature*. If guilt is the price to be paid for the illusion of control over nature . . . many people have seemed willing to pay it [p. 147].

RELIGIOUS GUILT AND SPIRITUAL PESSIMISM

Albert Einstein was once asked what the most important question was that human beings needed to answer. He replied, "Is the universe a friendly place or not?" If we believe in original sin or subscribe to a literal interpretation of God's punishment of Adam and Eve, then no matter how closely we may have examined our conscience, there is always room for doubt about the safety of our soul and the ultimate "friendliness" of the universe to "sinners." The state of helplessness created by that doubt gives rise to what I call spiritual pessimism, an existentially helpless position that is akin to, but much deeper than, psychological pessimism.

The central tenet of spiritual pessimism is: "This bad thing happened because God is punishing me for my sins." From this standpoint, illness or any crisis is the final proof of our unworthiness (either personal or as an entire race due to Adam's first sin). If psychological pessimism says, "This bad thing is all my fault, I mess up everything I do, and it's the story of my life," spiritual pessimism is worse still. The logic of spiritual pessimism goes this way: "This bad thing is all my fault, it is proof that I am unforgivable, and I am in for an eternity of suffering." Spiritual pessimism is the ultimate statement of fear because our very soul is in mortal danger.

I was on a talk show in Denver once when the host invited callers to phone in with their greatest fear. One man, nearly in tears, told us that he was absolutely terrified of an eternity in hell. I asked him gently, with the understanding that he might not want to discuss it publicly, what terrible thing he had done that he should fear hell. His answer was a true definition of spiritual pessimism. "Nothing that I can think of. But we're all sinners, and we're all going to burn. You have to be some kind of great saint—at least as good as Mother Teresa—to be saved. So how can I enjoy my life when I know what's going to happen to me? I worry about it every day."

Spiritual pessimism is closely tied to the low self-esteem that underlies chronic psychological helplessness. Regardless of what we were taught in Sunday school, we formulate our own idea of whether God is forgiving or punitive based on whether we felt psychologically safe or unsafe growing up, since God and parents are both larger-than-life authority figures with life-or-death power over us as children. The more frightened we were as children, the more religious guilt we are likely to feel as adults. And regardless of how we may intellectually commit ourselves to the optimistic view that bad events are invitations to insight and personal growth, if we have not done the psychological work of healing the frightened inner child, we are likely to remain emotionally convinced that we deserve God's wrath.

Psychologists Peter Benson and Bernard Spilka studied descriptions and definitions of God as given by Catholics and related it to their self-esteem. Even though the 128 people studied had identical religious education, their concepts of God differed markedly. The researchers found that people with high self-esteem—those who liked and trusted themselves—had loving, accepting images of God. Those with low self-esteem—guilty, pessimistic people—had punitive, rejecting images of God. The human tendency to view God as a projection of ourselves—literally made in our own image—is a serious trap for the guilty, whose separation from love occurs on every level, including separation from the Self, separation from others, and separation from God.

THE SHADOW OF SPIRITUAL PESSIMISM

Many of us hold onto a mask of spiritual security, thinking consciously that we're part of a safe universe as long as we abide by certain moral precepts, while we unconsciously hide our fear of divine punishment away in our shadow. But just as we project our psychological shadows on other people, seeing in them what is too scary or distasteful to see in ourselves, we also project our spiritual shadows.

Many years ago, in our "hippie" days, my husband, Myrin, and I had a dispute with our landlord and his wife, who seemed to distrust us on the basis of our long hair. We began to understand that we had become a screen for the projection of their shadow material when they took us to small claims court. While the hearing was meant to resolve the question of who should pay for the tank of oil delivered after we were evicted on short notice, the roots of their concern went much deeper. The landlords told the judge that our pet guinea pig, "Squeaky," was part of a fictitious rabbit colony kept in the cellar by "two crazy medical scientists" for experimental purposes!

The judge was quite amused and ended the affair by having us split the cost of the oil and ordering them to return a ladder, a vacuum cleaner, and a few other items that they had confiscated from us as we moved out. Mowing the lawn of our new home for the first time, Myrin broke his leg when the rotor blades kicked up a piece of scrap metal that had been hidden in the grass. When the landlord appeared at our new home to return the items a few days later, his wife spied Myrin's cast. "Aha," she cried, projecting her religious guilt and spiritual pessimism onto Myrin, "God is punishing you for your sins!" The old war cry of Bea Arthur as Maude, "God will get you for this!," is not so funny when people really believe it.

NEW AGE PHILOSOPHY AND SPIRITUAL PESSIMISM

The pervasive spiritual pessimism and religious indoctrination that often block authentic psychological and spiritual growth have resulted in a movement away from organized religion. The question is: Where are people moving to? What *can* we believe in? Since the mid-1950s, when Aldous Huxley wrote about the consciousness-expanding properties of peyote in his classic work *The Doors of Perception*, cultural interest in spiritual experience, as opposed to religious doctrine, has grown. Huxley quotes the poet William Blake: "If the doors of perception were cleansed, every thing would appear to man as it is, infinite."

The desire for that infinite experience while still in the body led to widespread experimentation with psychedelic drugs in the 1960s and early 1970s. Such drugs had been used for millennia in the religious rites of different cultures to open the doors of perception. But when used indiscriminately in a nonsacramental fashion by people unfamiliar with their effects and with no sacred frame of reference in which to appreciate their experience, results were haphazard. Some people had classical mystical experiences of light and splendor, returning from their "trips" in the supernal realm with the commitment to live life more fully and lovingly. Others had brief flashes of cosmic consciousness and returned with the arrogant notion that they were "in the know," while the rest of humanity was still steeped in ignorance. Yet others found themselves in dangerous backwaters of consciousness, where their own personal dragons became magnified; defenseless against them, they experienced true psychotic terror.

Even people who had mystic experiences on these drugs realized that they were just temporary glimpses into a realm that had to be reached some other way—the long way. There are no shortcuts to the intense inner work of self-discovery that leads to lasting psychological healing and the spiritual growth that accompanies it. The legacy of the psychedelic era was a renewed interest in the perennial philosophy and the age-old techniques of achieving wisdom, including meditation and contemplation. This renewal of interest resulted in an influx of Eastern philosophy and metaphysics into our Western culture. This influx, accompanied by a potpourri of other consciousness-expanding philosophies and techniques, which range from computerized technological systems for inducing brain-wave changes to channeling, are collected under the rubric "New Age."

Carl Jung, himself a serious student of Eastern mysticism, warned of the pitfalls of trying to export the beliefs of one culture to another whose psychology and metaphors were so different. He believed there were bound to be misunderstandings and misuses of the philosophy and its techniques. In a paper published in the *American Journal of Psychiatry* in 1985, coauthored by psychiatrist Ilan Kutz, Herbert Benson, and myself after we founded the Mind/Body Clinic together, Kutz points to Jung's ambivalence:

> Even Jung, who was better acquainted with mystical philosophy and in particular with Eastern thought, was ambivalent about its use. On the one hand he believed that Eastern "methods and philosophical doctrines (that) have been developed simply put all Western attempts along these lines into the shade." On the other hand, he was adamant about the irrelevance and misuse of Eastern teaching by Westerners: "People will do anything, no matter how absurd, in order to avoid facing their own souls. They will practice yoga and all its exercises, observe a strict regimen of diet, learn theosophy by heart, or mechanically repeat mystic texts from the literature of the whole world—all because they cannot get on with themselves and have not the slightest faith that anything useful could ever come out of their own souls."

Were Jung alive today to witness the so-called New Age Movement and its attempt to integrate Eastern mysticism and metaphysics into Western culture, he would see that the integration of East and West has indeed produced mixed results. There is no way to "package" Eastern thought for simple consumption in the way that Westerners are used to learning. Trained preferentially to memorize theorems and solve problems, the Western mind is ill-equipped for emptying the mind of concepts and waiting in Silence for experience. If experience does come, we want to own and label and categorize and file that experience away for future reference. We want to know what it *means*. Easterners are less concerned about meaning. To be is quite enough.

The attempted translation of Eastern thought is further impeded by the poverty of the English language. Hindu scripture, for example, is written in Sanskrit, a language rich in distinctions of meaning; its words convey an immediacy of experience unknown in English. Sanskrit contains hundreds of words that distinguish between different states of consciousness for which there are no English translations. Serious students of metaphysics realize the ancient principle that "the more you know, the more you realize how much you don't know." A little knowledge can be a dangerous thing if we think it is the whole truth. The Western mindset practically guarantees this premature desire to know the whole "truth."

As expected, enormous misconceptions and oversimplifications have arisen in New Age thinking. The classic misconception is the rather grandiose notion that "you create your own reality." While we certainly participate in creating our own reality, nowhere in Eastern thought is there a shred of evidence to support the notion that we are the sole authors of our own destiny.

The irony of this misconception, as we will see, is that while New Age philosophy grew out of a need to shuck off the chains of guilt and helplessness, "you create your own reality" is actually a warmed-over version of Western spiritual pessimism. We have projected the shadow of spiritual pessimism onto Eastern thought and therefore see what was never intended. The danger of the you-create-your-own-reality doctrine is that while, on the surface, it seems to offer new freedom to explore deeper wisdom grounded in the spiritual richness of the millennia, it is something quite different. In fact, it has replaced the iron chains of original sin with a set of golden chains that seem alluring but are no less a prison.

NEW AGE GUILT

> Ever since Shirley MacLaine went out on a limb and described her newfound spiritual powers, the slogan "we create our own reality" has become something of a self-help panacea. Clearly, a strong sense of personal empowerment offers a healthy alternative to a passive fatalism about life, a point convincingly argued by Yale surgeon Bernie Siegel in his bestselling book *Love, Medicine and Miracles*. However, in recent years a more extreme interpretation has taken hold in the alternative health field, a belief that we are personally responsible—on a conscious or unconscious level—for everything that happens to us.
>
> —"Editorial Comment," *New Age Journal*, September/October 1988 [p. 50]

The editors of *New Age Journal* go on to mention that these ideas are touted in a plethora of self-help books, including Louise Hay's surprise best-seller *You Can Heal Your Life*.

> Hay, who says she used this philosophy to cure her own cancer, holds that "we are each 100 percent responsible for all of our experiences." This unqualified assessment of human healing potential, apparently based on interpretations of metaphysical ideas such as karma and reincarnation, would be an understandable comfort to those facing serious illness—unless, of course, they fail to think themselves well.

Failure to think yourself well and the erroneous philosophy behind that notion creates what psychological/metaphysical scholar Ken Wilber refers to as New Age guilt, a concept that he and his wife, the late Treya Killam Wilber, developed more than a theoretical interest in. Before she passed on early in 1989, Treya had lived with breast cancer since their honeymoon in 1984. A 1988 interview with Ken and an article by Treya in *New Age Journal* called "Do We Make Ourselves Sick?" prompted the editorial comments cited above.

Ken Wilber is a serious, lifelong student of Eastern philosophy and Western psychology who has authored eleven books and hundreds of articles on consciousness and psychology, including the much-acclaimed *Spectrum of Consciousness*, which earned him a comparison to William James in terms of the scope and depth of his knowledge. Wilber is also an outspoken iconoclast with an acerbic wit. In the interview, Wilber attacks the you-create-your-own-reality notion as "narcissistic and grandiose." He laments:

> What the new agers managed to do, with regard to diseases physical in origin, was to not just misinterpret them as psychological in origin . . . but to go one step higher and interpret these diseases as spiritual in origin, as "lessons" you are giving yourself. . . . [They] say things like, "Well, what are you trying to teach yourself with this disease?" You might have, say, eye cancer, and they'll say, "What are you trying to avoid seeing?" Or you might have a broken leg and they'll say, "Why are you avoiding standing up for yourself?"

The psychology behind the uncritical acceptance of the you-create-your-own-reality doctrine and its illness-as-metaphor corollary is no different from what led fifth-century Christians to accept Augustine's doctrine of original sin. It seems to offer us a permanent cure for helplessness. What we create we can uncreate. We have power. If we fail, it is at least our own failure. Guilt, as Pagels reminds us, is preferable to helplessness.

Pessimistic people, because of their underlying helplessness, are at great risk. They are prone to confusing *responsibility* for learning to live well with an illness with *blame* for having caused it. Illness is seen as a failure, and the illusion of power is purchased by the attitude that we can cure what we have caused. Sometimes we can cure our bodies, but sometimes we can't. The idea that our bodily state is a simple reflection of our psychological or spiritual state is a dangerous and prevalent misunderstanding. Even great saints and enlightened beings get sick and die. Some die young and some die very old. Does the length of their life have any correlation with "how good" they were? They die from heart attacks and they die from cancer—the two leading causes of death in our society. And they don't die because God is punishing them, or some lesson has gone unlearned, or because they didn't meditate well enough.

I once came into a Mind/Body group with a cold, and some members reacted as if they'd caught the Pope in a brothel. How could I, who meditate, possibly catch cold? I got several questions like "Have you been very stressed lately?" and "What did you do to create this cold?" And I got comments like, "This cold is God's way of telling you to slow down."

Well, it certainly does help to listen to your body's messages. We do sometimes get sick from stress or fatigue, and illness can be a powerful message to do something differently. As you know, it has been an important teacher for me. But I also know that occasional colds are an occupational hazard for parents with school-age children and that it is quite possible to get one even if you're not stressed, depressed, or in need of rest! The same thing applies to cancer and every other illness. Genetics and environment are powerful factors that must not be ignored. If you breathe enough vinyl chloride, you will get liver cancer, no matter how optimistic you are. But because cancer is a frightening disease that epitomizes the loss of control for many of us, it's no wonder that we try to seek comfort in theories about why we get it. In pinning down the reasons, we think we can make ourselves safe.

Another facet of New Age guilt is the idea that illness is the fruition of past karma, an idea that takes the crime and punishment motif of Judeo-Christian spiritual pessimism and puts it in misunderstood Eastern wrappings. Karma refers simply to the law of nature that says that for every action there is an equal reaction, since energy is neither created nor destroyed but just changes forms. The lifeforce—the energy of creation—is always moving and assuming different configurations. In other words, if you throw a rubber ball against the floor, using muscular energy, it will bounce back and free the equivalent amount of energy as sound and heat. If you put out energy as anger, depending on the characteristics of the system it's added to, you might get anger back, or it may be transmuted into laughter, wisdom, sulking, love, violence, high blood pressure, or heartburn. This is cause and effect. It isn't a value judgment, it's just a natural law, like gravity.

If we ignore our shadow and keep making the same mistake time and time again, naturally we will experience our karma, the fruits of our actions, as some form of suffering. This does not mean, however, that everything that happens to us is "karmic" and that our karma is the complete cause of our joy or sorrow. A lung cancer that results from thirty years of smoking three packs of cigarettes daily is the fruit of our physical actions, perhaps aided in some small measure by sociological and behavioral factors. Even if a particular cancer is karmic, in the sense that it has to do with the fulfillment of energies that have accompanied our soul through different incarnations, we are in a poor position to understand what those forces are. As in the remarkable story of Brian Weiss's infant son, perhaps one person's illness is really an act of service for another person. We can't really say why things happen because we simply do not know. Attempts to do so may make us feel less helpless, but they are likely to create either guilt or a dangerous fantasy of omnipotence.

While we participate in creating reality, Eastern philosophy actually states that the human desire to believe that we create our own reality is one of the three *malas*—erroneous ideas that keep a person bound to the ego and unable to recognize the Self. The Shiva Sutras, a wisdom book from the ninth century, describes the karma mala as the attitude that keeps us in ignorance by preventing us from understanding and taking responsibility for the fruits of our action, thus stifling new action. Its origin is said to be in the "lack of awareness that Shiva (a form of the Divine Consciousness) is the only real agent or doer."

The challenge of our current age is to root out the personal and cultural misconceptions that keep us bound to repeating the same erroneous patterns over and over again. To do so, we must work toward a new model of psychological and spiritual health that will pay dividends in increased physical health. A starting point is the recollection of those traditions that speak of spiritual optimism in a familiar voice that can help us either to maximize the use of our own religious tradition as a conduit to the spiritual or to find an individual expression of spirituality in which we can grow.

ORIGINAL SIN OR ORIGINAL BLESSING? TRADITIONS OF SPIRITUAL OPTIMISM

The Dominican priest Matthew Fox has been a very outspoken critic of the Roman Catholic church and its doctrine of original sin, which poisoned the optimistic legacy of Christ and created the fallacy of spiritual pessimism. In *Original Blessing*, he reviews those traditionally optimistic aspects of religious doctrine that Augustine chose to turn away from. Fox chronicles the life-affirming, creation-centered spirituality that has been part of Western religious tradition since the ninth century B.C., when the psalms were written, and that was part of Eastern tradition for many centuries prior. He explains the perennial philosophy as it is present in Christianity, presenting the truly universal viewpoints of the great Christian mystics, including Julian of Norwich, Hildegard of Bingen, Francis of Assisi, Meister Eckhart, and many others.

Fox contrasts the original celebratory theology that sees life as a blessing with the much newer Augustinian fall/redemption theology that casts man into the role of a sinner, fallen from grace and in need of redemption by baptism from the moment of birth. He speaks passionately of religion being "out of touch with its sources of wisdom," and calls for the church to let go of its outdated, dualistic paradigm of original sin and conditional redemption that separates the Creator from the creation. According to Fox, on his deathbed Erich Fromm asked the central question that we have been considering in this book: "Why is it that the human race prefers necrophilia to biophilia?" In other words, why do we choose to say no to life, rather than yes. Fox answers:

> Western civilization has preferred love of death to love of life to the very extent that its religious traditions have preferred redemption to creation, sin to ecstasy, and individual introspection to cosmic awareness and appreciation. Religion has failed people in the West as often as it has been silent about pleasure or about the cosmic creation, about the ongoing power of the flowing energy of the Creator, about original blessing. . . . What has been most lacking in society and religion in the West for the past six centuries has been a Via Positiva, a way or path of affirmation, thanksgiving, ecstasy.
>
> —*Original Blessing* [p. 33]

Fox's theological concept of the Via Positiva is a statement of spiritual optimism, the idea that life is to be celebrated, not feared, because God created a universe out of loving-kindness with the purpose of teaching loving-kindness. It is a theology of love rather than fear, of wholeness rather than fragmentation, of eternal wisdom, love, and growth rather than of sin, punishment, and death.

While Fox has approached healing as a theologian, similar conclusions can be drawn from psychology. For example, most first-year psychology students can cite B. F. Skinner's findings that punishment is an effective way to change behavior, but usually not in the desired direction. Many parents have found the same thing. If you punish a child who doesn't do her homework, it rarely creates the desire to learn. Instead, it encourages anger, hatred, distrust, lying, and rebellion—in short, fear. On the other hand, reward and praise are very effective ways to change behavior. In a much-publicized study, teachers were told that their incoming classes had been tested for academic potential. They were given a list of students, actually chosen at random, as the likely high achievers. At the end of the year, those children had indeed met the teacher's expectations, since their efforts were preferentially recognized and rewarded.

Encouragement, recognition, and love lead to growth. Fear and punishment lead to helplessness, anxiety, depression, low self-esteem, loss of will, poor health, and the development of a false self. They lead to the syndrome of unhealthy guilt that develops in so-called dysfunctional families where the parents themselves have low self-esteem and cannot form authentic, nurturing interpersonal bridges with their children. In 1988, the Catholic church reacted to Matthew Fox's outspoken views by demanding that he observe a year of silence. Fox agreed to the year of silence after rebutting the church publicly by comparing it to a dysfunctional family. Psychologically, Fox was right on target. At the risk of sounding sacrilegious, why would we assume that God was less intelligent than B. F. Skinner when He designed the plan for our reunion with the Divine? Why would He use fear to teach love, promising punishment and damnation for the valuable mistakes we make along the hero's journey to the Grail of compassion?

THE PRODIGAL SON— A PARABLE OF SPIRITUAL OPTIMISM

Just as the story of Snow White serves as a blueprint for the healing of unhealthy guilt and psychological pessimism, the New Testament story of the Prodigal Son provides a parallel blueprint for healing spiritual pessimism. This gentle parable speaks to our proper relationship with a nurturing God and answers the central question of how He deals with our mistakes.

Jesus told the story of the Prodigal Son in a particular context. In Luke 15, the Pharisees were trying to impugn Jesus's integrity by accusing him of spending too much time with prostitutes and tax collectors, the big sinners of biblical times. Jesus replied with compassion, explaining that God's pleasure is in the return of such "lost sheep." After all, why preach to those who are already in connection with the Divine? He then offered the story of the Prodigal Son as an archetypal statement and promise of God's love and forgiveness and their outpouring to the sinner in the form of grace.

The story is a very simple one. A man had two sons. The younger one asked for his portion of their inheritance and ran off to a foreign land where he squandered it on wine, women, and riotous living. The older boy, meanwhile, stayed faithfully by his father's side, tilling the soil. Eventually the younger son ran out of money and, to make things worse, there was a famine in the land where he'd gone. He got a job feeding pigs, but he was so hungry that he would gladly have eaten the pig swill. Finally coming to his senses, he realized that even his father's servants had a better life than he did. He realized the error of his ways and decided to go home, apologize for his wrongdoing, and hope that his father would take him in at least as a hired hand.

When he was still some distance away, his father spotted him and ran out to meet him, greeting him with heartfelt hugs and kisses. The son apologized, admitting his mistakes, and was instantly forgiven. His father then had the servants bring his son the finest clothes and kill the fatted calf to make a banquet in his honor.

The faithful son was out in the fields during the homecoming. As he came back to the house, he heard music and the sound of dancing. Asking one of the servants what was happening, he found out that the party was for his brother, who had come home "safe and sound." At first he was angry and refused to go to the celebration, asking his father why in all his years of loyalty a calf had never been slaughtered for him so that he could have a party with his friends. Why was this done instead for his ne'er-do-well brother who "has devoured thy living with harlots"? The father lovingly explained that the faithful son had always been with him, and that everything he had was his. But "thy brother was dead and is alive again; and was lost and is found."

This story is a great psychospiritual teaching about love, forgiveness, and grace. Not knowing any better, we separate ourselves from the Source of Love and soon enough begin to suffer because we are cut off from our sustenance—we are literally starving. Suddenly we come to our senses and see that we have sinned (we have separated ourselves from love by our actions). Admitting what we have done (owning our shadow), we repent (we are sincerely sorry for our mistake), and we ask for forgiveness (to return home). Since this is God's greatest pleasure—to give us the

Kingdom—He is on the lookout for our desire to return and races right out to meet us, so delighted that he bestows his grace upon us and gives us all the good things of His kingdom. We die to our old ignorant self and are reborn to a new wise Self as the result of our adventure. The grace of working out our psychological integration attracts the grace that leads to spiritual integration.

THE UNION OF PSYCHOLOGICAL AND SPIRITUAL WISDOM

The false self evolved to protect us from the helplessness and fear of childhood, but as adults it prevents us from coming into our psychological and spiritual fullness. As long as we live with the erroneous presumption that we can exist with our good on one side of the wall and our "badness" sealed away in the shadow, we sacrifice any possibility of living a whole, authentic life. Creativity cannot flourish when our inner kingdom is divided against itself. Life becomes dry and barren. This is the psychological setting for Wolfram's Grail legend, as Joseph Campbell explains to Bill Moyers in *The Power of Myth*, the book that was produced out of the conversations that were edited into the PBS series of the same name.

> *Campbell*: The theme of the Grail romance is that the land, the country, the whole territory of concern has been laid waste. It is called a wasteland. And what is the nature of the wasteland? It is a land where everybody is living an inauthentic life, doing as other people do, doing as you're told, with no courage for your own life. That is the wasteland. . . .
>
> *Moyers*: And the Grail becomes?
>
> *Campbell*: The Grail becomes the—what can we call it?—that which is attained and realized by people who have lived their own lives. The Grail represents the fulfillment of the highest spiritual potentialities of the human consciousness.

Campbell goes on to explain how the Christian Grail King was wounded in a joust with a pagan warrior and why his kingdom became a wasteland.

> They both level their lances at each other, and they drive at each other. The lance of the Grail King kills the pagan, but the pagan's lance castrates the Grail King. What that means is that the Christian

> separation of matter and spirit, of the dynamism of life and the realm of the spirit, of natural grace and supernatural grace, has really castrated nature. And the European mind, the European life, has been, as it were, emasculated by this separation. And then what did the pagan represent? He was a person from the suburbs of Eden. He was regarded as a nature man, and on the head of his lance was written the word "Grail." That is to say, nature intends the Grail. Spiritual life is the bouquet, the perfume, the flowering and fulfillment of a human life, not a supernatural virtue imposed upon it.
>
> —*The Power of Myth* [pp. 196–97]

Campbell is saying, in effect, that nature intends the Via Positiva, that the material and spiritual meet in that joy. In living a full, self-aware life, when we are in touch with all of our instincts, rather than denying them as unholy, spiritual life arises like a flower from our psychological wholeness. They are one and the same thing.

Christianity was not always out of touch with nature and the wisdom that comes from knowledge of our natural instincts. An early form of Christianity called gnosticism derives from the Greek term *gnosis*, which Elaine Pagels defines as insight, or the intuitive process of knowing oneself. In her award-winning book *The Gnostic Gospels*, Pagels speaks of the intersection of psychological and spiritual wisdom, stating that "to know oneself, at the deepest level, is simultaneously to know God."

The Gnostic Gospels describes the history of gnosticism and some of the contents of the Nag Hammadi manuscripts, a remarkable collection of thirteen leather-bound papyruses and some loose papers that were found in the upper Egyptian desert in 1945, when a farmer accidentally unearthed a large earthenware jar that had lain buried for more than 1,600 years. The papyruses contained more than fifty manuscripts written at the time of the New Testament gospels and then translated from Greek to Coptic, the common Egyptian language of that time. Some of the manuscripts were gospels of Jesus's other disciples. There is even a Gospel of Mary Magdalene. Several of the documents claim to contain Jesus's secret teachings to the disciples—wisdom not intended for the masses.

Pagels describes the process by which the early church consolidated its doctrine, accepting some writings for inclusion in what became the New Testament and declaring others heretical, including those that we now refer to as the gnostic gospels. Gnostics, however, viewed themselves as mainstream Christians, not heretics. They differed from the church in believing that spirituality was an inner experience, not an intellectual doctrine. This view, naturally, didn't lend itself to the hierarchical structure of the church, in which doctrine had to be taken as a matter of faith.

Many of the teachings of Jesus and the parables preserved in the gnostic manuscripts are remarkably similar to those in the New Testament. Some are distinctly different. I was particularly excited by those teachings that stress the importance of the self-knowledge so central to gnosticism. In the gnostic gospel of Thomas, Jesus tells his disciples that the Kingdom of God is not a place but a consciousness existing both within us and beyond us. He goes on to explain that, without self-knowledge, we cannot realize the Kingdom: "Rather, the kingdom is inside of you, and it is outside of you. When you come to know yourselves, then you will become known, and you will realize that it is you who are the sons of the living father. But if you will not know yourselves, you will dwell in poverty and it is you who are that poverty."

The disciples then ask Jesus how they should get to the Kingdom: "Do you want us to fast? How shall we pray? Shall we give alms? What diet shall we observe?"

Jesus answers: "*Do not tell lies, and do not do what you hate* for all things are plain in the sight of heaven [italics added]."

These simple spiritual instructions for being truthful to oneself and honoring one's instincts and wishes absolutely delighted me. They are sound psychological advice for dismantling the false self and beginning to live an authentic life. When the disciples asked Jesus how he would be revealed to them—a question that really relates to how we will find the Inner Christ, the Inner Self—his answer was also profoundly psychologically healing:

> When you disrobe without being ashamed and take up your garments and place them under your feet like little children and tread on them, then (will you see) the son of the living one, and you will not be afraid.
>
> —"*The Gospel of Matthew,*" The Nag Hammadi Library

What better description could we have of taking off our masks, trampling them with the exuberance of the Natural Child, and taking pride in being who we are?

SPIRITUALLY OPTIMISTIC TRANSFORMATIONS

In reclaiming the wisdom traditions of spiritual optimism, like the gnostics, we must be prepared to be transformed by the wisdom, not merely informed by it. Wisdom that remains in the mind as an idea, rather than becoming incorporated into the tapestry of who we are, cannot change us. It just sits there in the concept file. Such religious concepts can, in theologian Huston Smith's words, "immunize us against" spiritual experience. We become like the college professor who went to visit a Buddhist monk. Holding out his tea cup to be filled, the professor was shocked when the monk continued to pour tea until the cup overflowed. "Why did you do that?" sputtered the professor. The Zen monk smiled kindly, "Your mind is like that cup. It is so full of concepts that there isn't room for any wisdom."

When wisdom transforms us, it becomes alive by joining with our personal history and showing us something new about ourselves, something that leads us to greater freedom and joy of being. Any good story or parable that is archetypal will do that if we will throw out our concepts about what the story is supposed to mean and inquire into what it means to *us*. Because we are literally new each day, each moment, as the contents of our experience combine in endless ways, these stories can reveal themselves freshly and newly in each reading. Our comprehension of them expands as our psychological self-awareness deepens. And our psychological self-awareness deepens as we read them once again.

Let's consider the Adam and Eve story again, using Joseph Campbell as our guide. Campbell points out that the story of Adam and Eve is not unique to the Old Testament but occurs as an archetypal story in many unrelated cultures. In *The Power of Myth*, he tells the creation story of the Bassari people of West Africa. Their version of Genesis begins when their God, Unumbotte, makes a human being and names it Man. Next he makes an antelope and then a snake. He sets the two animals to pounding the earth and then gives them seeds to plant. One day the animals, who are hungry, wonder why they shouldn't eat the fruit. Then Man and his wife do take the fruit and eat of it. At this point, Unumbotte descends from above and asks who ate the fruit. The couple reply that they did, but that it was the snake who made them do it.

Campbell explains that the snake is the symbol of regenerated life, throwing off the old and becoming new, just as the snake does when it sheds its skin. In the *Power of Myth*, Campbell says,

> Sometimes the serpent is represented as a circle eating its own tail. That's an image of life. Life sheds one generation after another, to be born again. The serpent represents immortal energy and consciousness engaged in the field of time, constantly throwing off death

> and being born again. There is something tremendously terrifying about life when you look at it that way. And so the serpent carries in itself the sense of both the fascination and the terror of life [p. 45].

In this light, Adam, Eve, and the Serpent were participating in the evolution of consciousness rather than setting the fall of man into motion. According to Elaine Pagels, certain of the Gnostic Christians likewise suggested that:

> The story was never meant to be taken literally but should be understood as spiritual allegory—not so much *history with a moral* as *myth with meaning*. These gnostics took each line of the scriptures as an enigma, a riddle pointing to deeper meaning. Read this way, the text became a shimmering surface of symbols, inviting the spiritually adventurous to explore its hidden depths, to draw upon their own inner experience—what artists call the creative imagination—to interpret the story.
>
> —*Adam, Eve and the Serpent* [p. 64]

When the story of Adam and Eve is treated as a living myth with meaning, it reveals the hidden depths of wisdom in many concepts that have been preserved as the tenets of spiritual pessimism—concepts about good and evil, sin, repentance, judgment, and the devil. A wonderful form of meditation consists in reading an archetypal story like Adam and Eve and then sitting in silent meditation, just being with the breath. Then one begins to contemplate the story, to let it unfold in the Silence beyond the concepts, so that it begins to reveal itself as a living truth working through the metaphors and experiences of your own life. Let's look at some old, pessimistic religious beliefs in this new light.

Good and Evil

According to the Augustinian interpretation of the Adam and Eve story, Eve was the conduit through which evil came into the world, rather than a heroine who confirmed the gift of free will and was the purveyor of wisdom and new life. Evil was personified by the snake, the devil, a creation of God that somehow turned permanently against its creator. In other cultures, however, the snake is revered as a wisdom symbol.

A completely different interpretation of the story unfolds if its universal metaphors are explored rather than taken at face value. Archetypically, the garden of Eden is the setting for a creation story that explains how the unmanifest energy of God—the formless Silence before the creative Word is spoken—gives rise to the visible world. Every culture and every religion has its version of this tale. Central to every creation story, however, is the formation of the pairs of opposites involved in material creation. According to the first chapter of *Genesis*:

> In the beginning God created the heavens and the earth. The earth was without form and void, and darkness was upon the face of the deep; and the Spirit of God was moving over the face of the waters. And God said, "Let there be light," and there was light. And God saw that the light was good; and God separated the light from the darkness. God called the light Day, and the darkness he called Night. And there was evening and there was morning, one day.
>
> —*The Book of Genesis*, 1:1–3, Revised Standard Version

The first act of creation is separating the opposites: heaven and earth, light and dark, day and night. In time, we get an infinity of opposites—man and woman, me and you, young and old, sick and well, beautiful and ugly, good and evil. In this way, the temporal world comes into being from the eternal consciousness. When Adam and Eve ate the apple, they left the womblike state of Unity with the unmanifest and entered into the phenomenal world of time where good and evil are one more pair of necessary opposites.

When evil is viewed as a relativity, with the humble knowledge that we have very limited spiritual sight, it becomes part of the natural order of things. Was Judas evil because he betrayed Jesus to the Romans? After all, Jesus knew in advance who his betrayer would be, and he announced it publicly at the last supper. Judas had been chosen to play a certain role in the drama—was he evil for carrying out his appointed role or would it have been evil to refuse his lot? For, after all, without the darkness that Judas brought temporarily into the world, there would have been no death and resurrection of the cosmic Christ.

The big problem we get into by examining absolutist concepts of good and evil is that we get such a limited view of the big picture. We "see through a glass, darkly." In Isaiah, it is written, "I form the light and create the darkness: I make peace and create evil; I am the Lord that doeth all these things." Where, after all, in creation is God absent if the lifeforce is the very substance of everything that is? Is He present in light but absent in darkness? Present in joy but absent in suffering?

Eastern philosophies, as well as the mystic branches of Christianity, Judaism, and Islam tell us that the inner Kingdom, where we become one with the Self, is a plane of consciousness that transcends the pairs of opposites. People who have had near-death experiences say similar things. Apparently evil happenings are necessary cogs in the wheel of a much larger drama that can only be appreciated when we step out of the phenomenal world into a greater consciousness. The mystery of this is entirely beyond human conception. We cannot even entertain what this means from our perspective.

On a more mundane level, good and evil are easier to deal with. Good things are those that increase the amount of love in the world. Evil things are those that deny love and perpetuate fear—what we commonly call sins. Yet we must remember how the poet Wolfram began the telling of the Grail legend: "Every act has both good and evil results." As Campbell reminds us, the best we can do is lean toward the light. But, as we will see in the next chapter, it is precisely in those acts where evil wins out that we can learn most quickly about compassion and achieve our true selfhood.

The Devil

The emphasis many of us place on evil entities, the Lucifers and Darth Vaders of creation, serves a function similar to religious guilt. It seems to be an answer to our helplessness, an attempt to stop apparently bad things from happening. Why is there an AIDS epidemic? It's Satan's fault, and we let him in because we sinned. Why do human beings sin? The devil makes us do it. The devil is actually the repository for the collective shadow of human consciousness. Thanks to him, we can worry less about the evil in our own shadows and project it outside of ourselves. But the more we worry about the evil "out there," the less we will see and deal with it in ourselves. This is the real way that the "devil" leads us into sin.

The idea that Lucifer, the angel whose name means "light," turned against God and became evil is a story that appears in many cultures and lends itself to different interpretations. One of the most charming is the Islamic tale told by Bill Moyers during his interviews with Joseph Campbell. The angels were originally created to serve God, but when God created man and placed him a little higher in the heavens than the angels, the angels were reassigned to serve man. Lucifer "sinned" against

God when he refused to serve man because he loved God so much that he could not bear the parting. Cast into hell for disobedience, Lucifer sustained himself in joy by remembering the voice of his beloved God as he told him to go to hell! The Hindus likewise tell us that the "hells" of life are the times that we feel separated from Divine love. We can create heavens out of these situations if, like the Lucifer of the Islamic story, we remember God.

If we prefer to view evil as an absolute force, a dark power that creates more darkness like a cosmic black hole, we quickly run into a number of interesting problems. Do we conclude that God was not strong enough to contain what the ancient Hebrews called the "evil urge"? In this case, the devil becomes like a cosmic cancer, a piece of the Divine body that has turned on itself and threatens the universe with destruction. By analogy, this point of view suggests that any good we do—any light we bring into the world—might also spontaneously transform itself into darkness. This takes the "free" out of free will and abrogates choice. We could also assume that the devil was an intentional creation. In that case, we are left with two choices, either God created him for good purpose or God himself is evil.

Sin

The very word sounds scary, like the hiss of that serpent slithering somewhere in the garden. And it's hard for most people to think of sin without thinking of punishment. The two go together in religious guilt like bread and butter. But from a practical, optimistic standpoint, when love is life's final goal, sin is any thought or deed that reinforces the sense of unworthiness and isolation. Like the Prodigal Son, our sins are invitations to self-awareness and an occasion to experience forgiveness and reunion. Sins are not acts by which we can be sentenced to an eternity in hell or undergo some kind of "second death" in which our soul ceases to be.

Fear and the thoughts, actions, and judgments it creates separate us from our own Self, from other people, and from God. Sin is anything that separates us from joy and enthusiasm, from loving our neighbor as ourself, from feeling our connection to everything else in the universe. This applies to murder, rape, theft, and all types of violence, which can occur only when we think we are separate from the person or thing we are violating, when we have no compassion or sympathy with another human being. It also applies to nonactions—sins of omission—such as staying in a marriage or a job where we are victimized, belittled, or otherwise stifled. In these cases, we have no sympathy for ourselves.

Repentance

The Prodigal Son came to his senses and realized that his sins had separated him from his father. Not wishing to suffer any more, he admitted that he was wrong and was willing to take responsibility for the consequences of his acts. This is repentance. *Repentance is awareness*, recognition of a blind spot, acknowledging the shadow so that we will be free to make more life-affirming choices in the future. This process can be very painful, for loss of our idealized self-image, our mask, is often frightening and depressing. But without repentance there is no forgiveness. We cannot forgive ourselves, nor can we receive the forgiveness of other people or of God until we are aware of and willing to admit our mistakes.

Judgment

One of the most interesting things about the parable of the Prodigal Son is that it contains no element of judgment by God. The son judges himself by considering the consequences of the actions he chose, and he deduces that he made a wrong choice. He then exercises his free will and repents, setting the wheels of forgiveness into motion. If we could really believe that this story is true for all of us, we would be free from the oppressive fear of Divine punishment that fuels religious guilt.

I once had a patient, a kind and intelligent young professor named Jeff, who was a very rational man. Dying from leukemia, he began questioning whether there was a God, a judgment, or an afterlife, but then dismissed it all and went back to his lifelong position as an atheist who believed that life in all its forms is a biological accident. According to Susan, his wife, Jeff had a lot of fear as his body died and was in an agitated state for hours before he finally let go. His passing was most difficult for them both. And then a most remarkable and magnificent—what I used to call miraculous—event occurred. Several hours after Jeff's death, Susan was sitting alone in their living room when the air became suddenly electric and Jeff materialized as a full, lifelike vision. Like the other people who have such visions, Susan insisted, "It wasn't a hallucination. He was really there."

The vision lasted for several minutes while Jeff explained to his wife that he couldn't leave her with the mistaken thought that death was terrible and life was a biological accident. He described a complete "life-after-life" experience with all the usual components of a near-death experience, except that, if we're willing to believe Susan, in his case it was the real thing. Jeff described the usual sequence of moving out of a tunnel into an ineffable, indescribable, loving light that is completely accepting and feels like a homecoming. The light is intelligent, all-knowing, and *totally forgiving*. People who have these experiences themselves and live to talk about them report that they don't want to leave the light and return to life as we know it. But at some point they realize that they must, and that their earthly life is like a sojourn in a classroom whose lessons will lead to a more permanent reunion with the lifeforce.

In the presence of the light, many people experience an instantaneous life review, not so that some cosmic judge and jury can assign them eternal lodgings in heaven or hell, but to allow them to appreciate what they have learned and what remains to be learned from the most important standpoint. *Did your actions spread love or did they hurt people? Did you learn compassion?* Rather than an intellectual recollection of deeds, people report that the life review is centered on emotions, on feelings. The consequences of your actions as they affected other people—creating either love or fear—are revealed through the perspective of the people you interacted with, rather like the scene in which Scrooge is shown the impact of his behavior by the Ghost of Christmas Past. While this is occurring, people report being surrounded by the light of forgiveness and knowing that they are forgiven by God. The question is whether they can forgive themselves.

In *Heading Toward Omega*, Dr. Kenneth Ring's book about the meaning of the near-death experience, a young woman talks about her life review and the judgment:

> You are shown your life—and you do the judging. . . . It's the little things—maybe a hurt child that you helped or just to stop to say hello to a shut-in. Those are the things that are most important. . . . You have been forgiven all your sins, but are you able to forgive yourself for not doing the things you should have done and some little cheaty things that maybe you've done in life? Can you forgive yourself? This is the judgment.

Heaven and Hell

In an old story, a man dies and an angel ushers him into a gorgeously appointed room. There are bowls of steaming delicacies on the table, and the people are rosy-cheeked and well-fed. There are Jews and Christians, Buddhists and Moslems, atheists and agnostics, people of every race and religion, black and white, red and yellow, young and old. They're singing, hugging, laughing, and having a fine time. But, strangely, the spoons there are very long, too long for a person to feed himself. However, this just adds to the merriment because people are enjoying feeding one another and being cared for in return.

When the angel opens the door to the next room, there are the same velvet drapes, celestial music, sweet aromas, and bowls of steaming delicacies, the same mixture of sizes and shapes, religions and races. But there is no joy and no song, only screaming and groaning. The people there are sallow and sickly, wasting away from starvation, and consumed with anger and frustration, each trying fruitlessly to fit the spoon into his own mouth. This, explains the angel, is the difference between heaven and hell: compassion. If we have not learned to suffer with, we will suffer alone.

Heaven and hell are not places but states of mind. As John Milton wrote in *Paradise Lost*, "The mind is its own place, and in itself can make a heaven of hell, a hell of heaven."

The poet Kabir writes:

Friend, hope for the Guest while you are alive.
Jump into experience while you are alive!
Think . . . and think . . . while you are alive.
What you call "salvation" belongs to the time before death.

If you don't break your ropes while you are alive,
do you think
ghosts will do it after?

The idea that the soul will join with the ecstatic
just because the body is rotten—
that is all fantasy.
What is found now is found then.
If you find nothing now,

you will simply end up with an apartment in the City of Death.
If you make love with the divine now, in the next life
you will have the face of satisfied desire.

SUGGESTIONS FOR THE READER

1. Are you a spiritual optimist or a spiritual pessimist? Why? What are the concepts that create your optimism or pessimism? Do you really believe these concepts from experiencing their effect in your life, or are they just ideas that you adopted from someone else or from your religious upbringing?

2. Choose a wisdom parable like Adam and Eve, Wolfram's Grail legend, the Prodigal Son, or any myth that intrigues you. Use it for meditative contemplation.

PART THREE

Compassion: The Flower of Psychospiritual Growth

Listen, friend, listen to your heart
Hear compassion in the murmur of love
I Am That I Am
You Are That You Are

We are the light of world
saints and sinners
teachers and learners
the beloved and the reviled

revealed at last in magnificent splendor
in that magic moment when
seeing God in ourselves
We see Him also in each other.

—J. B.

CHAPTER EIGHT

Forgiveness

Writing for *Parabola Magazine*, P. L. Travers spins an enchanting tale of forgiveness staged in the dark, enchanted forest of our own unconscious. The heroine of this story is always dimly aware of a woman dressed in a long blue veil just at the edge of her awareness, always searching for something—never directly in her sight, yet never out of it either. In a sudden moment of decision, the lady in blue blocks her way and reaches out for the acknowledgment she has always wanted and needed:

> So we stood there facing each other, vibrant in the expectant stillness, the forest birdsong suddenly silent. Then she thrust a hand under her veil and drew it down from head to shoulder, her face emerging as a moon slips out from the edge of a cloud. . . . It was my face. . . . And I knew that I had always known . . . . "Forgive me," she said. "I am what I am." As she spoke her veil slithered to the ground revealing a white under-gown that was tucked and puckered and stained with living. And looking down, I saw that my own robe was equally tucked and puckered and stained. . . . The same face, the same garments, the other aspect of myself—and I had rejected it, believing, in my ignorance that I could go on my pilgrimage unshadowed and alone.
>
> —From "The Meeting," by P. L. Travers,
> *Parabola Magazine*, August 1987

Travers reminds us that we need our shadows and they need us. "How can one set out on the road to Heaven without taking note of the earth one treads on. . . . How could the Self perform its hero task without the Ego to contend with?" The final scene of this archetypal meeting in the woods captures the essence of psychospiritual healing in the grace-filled act of divine self-forgiveness:

> Arms wide, we bent toward each other. And a passing angel paused for a moment, standing imponderably on the air, to witness our embrace. "Wherever there are two, there are three!" He smiled at us benignly, "May that Third, the One that reconciles, unnameable, not to be seen or known, in mercy forgive you both."
>
> —From "The Meeting," by P. L. Travers, *Parabola Magazine*, August 1987

COMPASSION

The poetic images of this enchanting story trace the process of psychospiritual integration that is the hero's journey. When the split between mask and shadow is healed, and the Oneness of the Self revealed, the journey is complete and we claim the Grail that Campbell has defined as the flower of spiritual life, the attainment of compassion. In compassion, the state of *sympathy with*, or empathy, we voluntarily share in the experience—the suffering, the passion—of another person. At some level, we comprehend that we are not two, but one.

As we discussed in the last chapter, human beings have always looked for ways to understand suffering and hopefully to avoid it. But we cannot. Sickness, aging, and death are part of the nature of life. Twenty-five hundred years ago, the father of young Prince Gautama wanted to shield his child from suffering. Kept in the confines of the palace grounds, the prince's every desire was immediately fulfilled. But one day Gautama's curiosity overwhelmed him, and he commanded his charioteer to take him to the city. For the first time, he saw sickness, poverty, old age, and death. In that moment, he was overwhelmed by compassion. The suffering of others was his own suffering. The young prince immediately fled from the palace and took up a solitary life of contemplation, seeking the reasons for and the way of release from the suffering of human life. He became the Buddha.

The Buddha spoke of four Noble Truths, the first of which is that suffering is a universal fact of human life. The other three Noble Truths concern the origin of suffering, the cessation of suffering, and the Eightfold spiritual path of intentional, conscious living that leads beyond suffering. Central to Buddhist teachings, as to Christianity, is the practice of compassion. When Jesus was asked to summarize spiritual life, he was quite Buddhist in his reply. We should love God first—understand the ground of our being—and then we would love our neighbor as ourself. This is the Christian ideal of *agape*, compassionate love. In sharing the suffering of another, we participate in a mystery in which suffering is transformed into love.

The Buddhists believe that in every age an enlightened soul appears on earth to bring knowledge of God and thereby alleviate suffering. These compassionate beings, who voluntarily reenter the field of space and time to give their life for others, are called *bodhisattvas*. Jesus, for example, was a bodhisattva. As Joseph Campbell puts it in the *Power of Myth*:

> The Bodhisattva represents the principle of compassion, which is the healing principle that makes life possible. Life is pain, but compassion is what gives it the possibility of continuing. The bodhisattva is one who has achieved the realization of immortality yet voluntarily participates in the sorrows of the world. Voluntary participation in the world is very different from just getting born into it. That's exactly the theme of Paul's statement about Christ in his Epistle to the Philippians: that Jesus "did not think Godhood something to be held on to but took the form of a servant here on earth, even on to death on the cross." That's voluntary participation in the fragmentation of life [p. 112].

In recent years, Americans have begun to value the ideal of selfless service that is epitomized in the symbol of a bodhisattva. Charles Kuralt once did a television special called "Small Town America" that featured several very moving acts of compassion performed by ordinary citizens. What I remember best was a woman from the Midwest. During the Second World War, thousands of young GI's passed through her town on the train before going overseas. She organized the women in town, and they made sure that every boy had a last home-cooked meal before going to war. This is selfless service born of compassion, what Buddhists call *seva* and Christians call charity.

Dominique LaPierre's international best-seller *City of Joy* is the most moving true story of compassion that I have ever read. The book's title seems improbable at first, because the City of Joy is the name of one of the worst slums in Calcutta. Dwelling there is a young Polish priest, Stephen Kovalski, who gave up his comfortable middle-class life to share the vermin-infested hovels and scanty food of the city's poorest and most wretched inhabitants. The involuntary dwellers in the slum were no less remarkable than the priest, transforming misery into joy by the compassion they had for one another. In one scene, a leper named Anouar, in great pain because of gangrene, was creeping through the mud on a little tray with wheels, since his legs were reduced to stumps. Noticing a preoccupied look on Anouar's face, Kovalski stooped down to take his hand and ask what was wrong. Anouar replied, "Oh nothing, Stephan Daddah, I'm fine. But my neighbor, Säid, is not too good. You ought to come and see him. He's so ill he can't eat or sleep." Dominique Lapierre, who lived in the slum himself for a year and wrote the book out of that experience, continues: "The cripple creeping along in the filth asked nothing for himself. Worried only about his neighbor, he was the living message of the Indian proverb 'The hell with misery as long as we're miserable together.' "

FORGIVENESS

Forgiveness is the exercise of compassion and is both a process and an attitude. In the process of forgiveness, we convert the suffering created by our own mistakes or as a result of being hurt by others into psychological and spiritual growth. Through the attitude of forgiveness, we attain happiness and serenity by letting go of the ego's incessant need to judge ourselves and others. We will consider forgiveness as a process first, and then discuss it as an attitude later in the chapter. But first I would like to recall a story I told in *Minding the Body, Mending the Mind*, because it demonstrates my belief about forgiveness. The incident involved a young boy of color who leaned out the back window of his family's old car and made a vulgar gesture toward me for no apparent reason. It was easy to see that his behavior had nothing to do with me but must have been caused by pain created by societal or family concerns. Instead of adding to his pain, I mustered up all the love I could and beamed it out to him in a big smile. He suddenly began to smile in return, and we waved at one another until his car was out of sight. Forgiveness is not a self-righteous or Polyanna-like turning of the other cheek by which we condone anathema behavior. But if we can understand the deep pain from which hurtful actions inflicted on us arose, then we have suffered with the other person; we have been compassionate. In that act of compassion, we move out of the role of victim and see beyond their actions to the person who is acting. Forgiveness does not require us to become friends with, for example, an abusive parent, to care for them in their old age, or to do anything in particular. Forgiveness is a state of mind that may give rise to specific actions but is not defined by those actions.

Forgiveness toward ourselves is described beautifully in P. L. Travers's story, excerpted at the beginning of the chapter. It is a seeing beyond our own actions to the person who is acting. It is the acceptance of our shadow so that we can be whole. This requires the long, hard work of psychospiritual integration that we have been discussing in the first two parts of the book. Forgiveness requires awareness—the commitment to self-knowledge. Old hurts cannot be cancelled and undone, but these emotions can become the seeds of transcendence that allow healing to occur, whether we are the victim or the aggressor.

I have had the pleasure of working with many members of twelve-step programs, which derive considerable power from their emphasis on forgiveness. Many people in programs like Alcoholics Anonymous enter recovery with a heavy burden of healthy guilt for the suffering they have caused themselves and others. I was amazed and delighted to learn how they help one another face their healthy guilt and reach new levels of psychospiritual awareness through forgiveness. Remarkably, steps four through ten—seven of the twelve steps of recovery from addiction—deal directly with facing and growing from healthy guilt. The other five steps set the stage, support the effort, and encourage the final hero function of sharing one's learnings compassionately with other people in similar circumstances.

Milton, a man in his early sixties, was a new member of Alcoholics Anonymous struggling through the early stages of forgiveness when he came to me for help with angina. As he told me the history of his disease, I could see that he was very much in tune with his thoughts and feelings and their effect on his body. The squeezing chest pain that sent Milton for his nitroglycerine came from two sources: exercise, for which his heart muscle required more blood than his clogged coronary arteries could deliver; and remorse, which gripped his heart just as tightly.

When I asked about his guilt, Milton responded with honesty and insight. "I've got plenty to be guilty about, Joan. Thirty-some years of drinking touches a lot of lives. When I think about what my wife went through—my angry and unpredictable moods, the time I lost my job because of the booze, having to raise the kids pretty much by herself—I was never really there for her. Then there are our two boys, smart kids and one of them didn't even finish college. Do you have any idea what it's like to have a father who's hardly there for you except to criticize?" Milton shook his head and wiped away a tear. "And that's just the beginning. I've made more mistakes than I could tell you about in ten more sessions."

Milton was at the beginning of the forgiveness process—facing the pain that motivates self-knowledge. He took a lot of comfort in the New Testament, particularly the stories about Mary Magdalene, whose great longing for forgiveness awakened her legendary love for Christ.

In the New Testament, there is a beautiful story about Mary Magdalene in the seventh chapter of the Gospel of Luke. Simon, one of the Pharisees, invites Jesus for supper. Mary Magdalene also comes, and Simon thinks to himself that Jesus couldn't possibly be a man of God or he would know what kind of despicable woman she was. Reading his thoughts, Jesus responds to Simon with a parable, asking him a question. "There was a certain creditor that had two debtors: the one owed five hundred pence, the other fifty. And when they had nothing to pay, he frankly forgave them both. Tell me, then, which of them will love him most?" Simon, of course, answered that the one with the biggest debt would be most grateful. Jesus responded that Mary Magdalene's sins, which were many, were forgiven because "she loved much: but to whom little is forgiven, the same loveth little."

THE TWO SIDES OF FORGIVENESS

In the equation of error, we're either debtors or creditors, the "mistaker" or the "mistaken," the aggressor or the victim. Like any pair of opposites, these are two sides of one coin. They need one another in order to exist and to allow forgiveness to manifest. There's a Buddhist idea, in fact, that suffering exists specifically to teach us compassion. This idea has helped me face my actions so that I could go on to forgive myself for the hurts I've caused other people and forgive them for the hurts they've caused me. We are all teachers to one another. Without error on someone's part, none of us would learn the lesson of compassion that forgiveness is.

As long as we continue to identify with one side of the coin exclusively—debtor or creditor—we remain psychologically one-up or one-down on the other person. Forgiveness requires us to give up our ideas of better and worse and to finally see ourselves as equals and colearners. This is a hard lesson when we've been hurt and our debtor seems unrepentant, but regardless of what they learn or don't learn in the process or how fast or slow they are at it, forgiveness is up to us. *Forgiveness is not conditional on someone else's behavior.* If we insist that it is, we cannot move out of the victim position. Holding onto being the victim is the surest way of staying stuck and blocking our healing.

The steps to forgiving ourselves and others are parallel six-step processes that may take quite some time to complete. If we manage to do it in a lifetime, in fact, and reach the state of enlightenment that is the final outcome of the process, we are much blessed. The object is not to hurry but to let things unfold, as they will, from your own intention to forgive.

THE STEPS TO FORGIVING OURSELVES

The steps are:

1. Take responsibility for what you did.
2. Confess the nature of your wrongs to God, yourself, and another human being.
3. Look for your good points.
4. Be willing to make amends where possible, as long as you can do this without harm to yourself or other people.
5. Look to God for help.
6. Inquire about what you have learned.

Step One: Taking Responsibility

The first step in the forgiveness process—taking responsibility—might be illustrated by a story that took place when I was sixteen years old and taking the family car out for only the third time. It was out of gas, so I pulled into a station. They must have been used to reckless drivers there because they protected their pumps with a barricade of red pipe fencing that I promptly crunched with my left rear fender. My mouth turned dry as dust, my palms poured sweat, and I was sure that my beating heart could be heard for blocks. What to do? I was afraid that if I told the truth I'd never get the car again, but, on the other hand, I didn't want to lie. I settled anxiously for the middle ground. Playing dumb. Maybe no one would notice, at least for a while.

I went to my room, where I obsessed endlessly over all the bad things that would certainly happen to me when my parents found out. That night I barely slept. Bright and early the next morning, my mother discovered the dent and asked me what I knew about it. I couldn't bear to admit the truth, so I lied. "Maybe someone backed into the car in the parking lot." That seemed to get me off the hook outwardly, but inwardly I felt worse than ever. Now I had two guilts to bear—the guilt of the accident and the guilt of hiding it.

It wasn't until years later, when it no longer seemed to matter, that I finally confessed to my father. The irony was that he had known all along. After all, he bought his gas at the same garage! Since he had already forgiven me, understanding both the problems of new drivers and the fear I had of confessing, he had let the episode pass. I was the one who was holding on, fearful of admitting my mistake. Many times the fear of punishment, or just looking bad, keeps us stuck in guilt the way I was. We know what we've done, but we don't acknowledge it.

In *Minding the Body, Mending the Mind*, I discussed other ways that we fail to take responsibility for our actions and feelings. Denial is a common one. What me? Anxious, angry, jealous, an addict of some sort? Never. I am beyond reproach (at least in that regard). Hiding from ourselves, pushing away the shadow and keeping it repressed in the unconscious, keeps us fragmented and fearful, afraid of the part of ourselves that we don't know. But until we've recognized our own hidden parts, how can we reown them and become whole again? Rationalization is another very common means of disowning responsibility. Why should I pay my fair share of the income tax? After all, they are only going to make bombs with it. Or why should I put in all this effort at work when other people goof off?

Taking responsibility for our actions and our mistakes is a necessary step toward self-knowledge because it leads to the inevitable question "Why?" Why did I do what I did? If we take the "why" behind intentional acts far enough, we will almost always meet fear—the "devil" that made us do it! With awareness of our fear, we become freer to make more loving choices in the future.

Step Two: Confession

Confession and forgiveness are a common ground where mind, body, and spirit meet. Holding onto dark, guilty secrets is similar to repressing trauma—it takes physiological work that leads to increased stress and illness. I was at a conference once where Dr. James Pennebaker presented studies on the health benefits of confession. His interest was first piqued by lie detector technicians who told him about all the birthday and Christmas cards they get from grateful prisoners who still remember the vast relief of confessing their crimes!

Pennebaker recounted the story of a man who had embezzled money from the bank where he worked. He was miserable, tormented by his guilt for six months, during which time he had a steady stream of colds, flus, and other illnesses. When he was finally called in for a lie detector test, he was naturally stressed out and anxious. But, as soon as he confessed, his body went into a profound state of relaxation, even though he had entered the test a free man and completed it a confessed embezzler who would go to jail.

Jung believed that confession was part of the deep religious longing of each person to reunite with the Source, and that it was a major contributor to the effectiveness of psychotherapy. Unless we belong to a church where the sacrament of confession is practiced, or to a twelve-step program where we can count on the love and support of others while we confess our addiction and the hurts it created, the therapist is often the first one to hear the dark secrets of our hearts. Jung wrote:

> To cherish secrets and hold back emotion is a psychic misdemeanor for which nature finally visits us with sickness—that is when we do these things in private. But when they are done in communion with others they satisfy nature and may even count as useful virtues. . . . There would appear to be a conscience in mankind which severely punishes everyone who does not somehow and at sometime, at whatever cost to his virtuous pride, cease to defend and assert himself, and instead confess himself fallible and human. Until he can do this, an impenetrable wall shuts him off from the vital feeling that he is a man among other men. This explains the extraordinary significance of genuine, straightforward confession—a truth that was probably known to all the initiation rites and mystery cults of the ancient world. There is a saying from the Greek mysteries, "Give up what thou hast, and then thou wilt receive."
>
> —*Problems to Modern Psychotherapy*, volume 16 [p. 58]

Step Three: Overcoming Depression by Looking for the Good

Confession to ourselves, to another human being, and to God in heartfelt prayer is a major step toward forgiveness. But there is a pitfall in confession. Serious depression can result from acknowledging the depth of problems caused by our own denial, greed, hatred, self-righteousness, or anger. We may catch a glimpse of the shadow and become terrified by it, immobilized by the fear that we are indeed great sinners, temporarily forgetting all our good points. But if we fall into the pit of depression, we won't be able to move forward. Rabbi Nachman, a Jewish tzaddik, or enlightened wiseman, who lived in the late 1700s and early 1800s, wrote of this in a wonderful treatise on forgiveness recently published with the title *Restore My Soul*:

> The essence is to remove from yourself every hint of the bitter blackness of depression. The fundamental reason why people are far from God is because of depression. They lose their morale, they come to despise themselves because they see the blemishes within themselves and the great damage which they do. In secret each one knows the soreness of his own heart and his private pain [p. 26].

But how can we remove depression over a mistake that has made us guilty, especially if we are already depressed by a chronically pessimistic attitude? In depression we see only our bad points. The cure, both according to modern cognitive therapists and to Rabbi Nachman, is to *look for the good points persistently*, even if the inner voices of darkness insist that we are evil. Nachman says:

> It is everyone's duty to search and search until he finds within himself some point of goodness. How is it possible that in all his days he never once fulfilled at least one precept or performed one good deed? But no sooner does he start examining this good which he did, then he begins to realize that even this good was "full of sores, there is no soundness in it" (Is. 1:6). The good was blemished and bound up with false motives. Still, somewhere in this little bit of good there must exist at least some "good points." Now the search must begin again. . . . This is the way for a person to find the goodness and merit in himself. He emerges from the scale of guilt and enters the scale of merit [pp. 25–26].

Step Four: Making Amends

Some mistakes are relatively easy to correct. A shoplifter who is seized with remorse can mail the money for the goods back to the store. But when a person rather than an institution has been hurt by our actions, we often need to communicate with him as part of making our amends. This means apologizing. A person who was overcome with anxiety when his friend got cancer and found himself unable to communicate and offer support can write a note, phone or visit, and apologize for the way that his fear blocked the expression of love. In facing the other person and letting them know that we understand what we did, we're sorry for it, and we hope that they can forgive us, we are repenting.

There are, however, instances where making amends creates fresh damage. If an old boyfriend who left you in the lurch suddenly showed up on your doorstep during the first years of your marriage, his attempts to release the old pain might create new problems for you. So, before making amends, think through the possible repercussions. If it is not possible to communicate with the person you hurt directly, do it as part of a meditation. After you calm yourself down, imagine that you are in a safe and familiar place. Then imagine inviting the person you have hurt into that place and have a conversation. Tell them you are sorry, and explain what happened. Listen to their reply. And then ask them to forgive you. End by forgiving yourself.

Step Five: Looking to God for Help

> He who approaches near to Me one span, I will approach to him one cubit; and he who approaches near to Me one cubit, I will approach near to him one fathom, and whoever approaches me walking, I will come to him running, and he who meets Me with sins equivalent to the whole world, I will greet him with forgiveness equal to it.
>
> —From the *Mishkat al-masabih*

Pain yearns for comfort. When we recognize how far we are from God, like the Prodigal Son we yearn to go home. When we are absolutely miserable, prayer is no longer a dry rote repetition. It becomes a living and vibrant cry for help. It becomes authentic. In pain we forget the "thee's" and "thou's" that keep us separated from God, and reach a new state of intimacy that comes from talking to God in our own way, saying what's in our heart. Some of the most magnificent prayers ever written, in fact, came from the pain of facing guilt and the intimacy with the Divine that it creates. This is what motivated King David to write the psalms.

The story of David's grievous sin and subsequent repentance is the subject of the eleventh chapter of the Second Book of Samuel in the Old Testament, and it's quite a story. Late at night, David got out of bed and went up on the roof for some air. While there, he happened to see the beautiful Bathsheba washing herself and was overcome with desire. He dispatched a servant to fetch her, and they made love. Bathsheba became pregnant with his child, and when she told him, David lost his judgment entirely. He shipped her husband, a loyal soldier named Uriah, off to the thick of battle, hoping he'd be killed at the front, which he was. When the mourning period was over, David and Bathsheba married. God then sent the prophet Nathan to David, who helped him face the enormity of what he had done. Shortly thereafter, when the son of the illicit liaison died in infancy, David's already troubled heart was broken.

David's guilt, heartache, and subsequent longing for reunion with God were the impetus he felt to write the psalms, a moving compendium of many different types of prayer. The psalms encompass all the emotions that come up in the long process of forgiveness—outpourings of pain, confession, and repentance. Prayers for strength and courage like the Twenty-third Psalm, "The Lord is my shepherd . . . ," are celebratory prayers of God's love, compassion, and the goodness of life. Reading the psalms is a great guide to forgiveness and a tremendous comfort when we realize that Jesus, the very embodiment of the teaching of forgiveness, ultimately arose from the House of David.

Later, David and Bathsheba had another son, who was King Solomon, reputedly the wisest man of all time. It is said that Solomon had a ring inscribed with the most important advice for human beings to remember. It said, "This too shall pass." These are good words to bear in mind during the time when one's inner pain is very great.

Step Six: Reflection: What Have I Learned?

Each time we hurt someone, admit it, and go through the steps for self-forgiveness, we learn something about ourselves that will help us function with more clarity and make better choices in the future. After all, we can't exercise free will when our vision is clouded with ghosts from the past that prevent us from seeing the present. The realization that our wrongs stemmed from fear, that they were in some way the action of a frightened child, teaches us to be compassionate toward ourself and spurs us on to heal the inner wounded child. And when we see that our own hurtful actions spring from fear, we can better understand that the actions of people who hurt us also spring from fear. This compassionate vantage point makes it easier to release ourselves from the chains of anger and resentment that can weigh on us so heavily when we are unable to forgive others.

THE STEPS TO FORGIVING OTHERS

Psychotherapist Robin Casarjian reads the following excerpt from a *Time* magazine article at her forgiveness workshops:

> The psychological case for forgiveness is overwhelmingly persuasive. Not to forgive is to be imprisoned by the past, by old grievances that do not permit life to proceed with new business. Not to forgive is to yield oneself to another's control. If one does not forgive, then one is controlled by the other's initiatives, and is locked into a sequence of action, a response of outrage and revenge. The present is overwhelmed and devoured by the past. Those who do not forgive are those who are least capable of changing the circumstances of their lives. In this sense, forgiveness is a shrewd and practical strategy for a person or a nation to pursue, for forgiveness frees the forgiver.

As this article states so clearly, one of the greatest causes of physical and emotional suffering is holding onto pain, refusing to let go because of our hurt. This was the sad case of George, a man who came to see me for help with bleeding ulcers that kept recurring despite his medications. George was a tall man, pale and thin. His curly hair was already gray, but bushy dark eyebrows framed his lonely, watery-blue eyes. As he shuffled slowly past me to take a chair, he looked much older than his fifty-five years, as if he were carrying the weight of the whole world on his shoulders.

Settling back against the chair, looking helpless and exhausted, George began to tell the story of his ulcers, weight loss, and sleeplessness. When I asked what was going on in his life when the ulcers started, a sudden fire blazed in his tired eyes, and he leaned forward with clenched fists.

His beautiful daughter, Rachel, "the light of his life," had married a gentile rather than a Jew. And he could not forgive her. George's wife went to the wedding, but he stayed home. Two years had passed, and he would not speak to his child, he had "cut her out" of his life. While George could acknowledge that his anger and hurt were literally eating his insides out, he insisted that he couldn't and wouldn't let go.

But what did George gain by holding on? When I asked him, all he could say was that his daughter would have to live her life in full knowledge of the pain her betrayal had caused. I asked him, "What about the pain *your* attitude is causing, George?" "I have a right," was the self-righteous reply, "but she had no right. She let down her people, and she let down her parents."

The Buddha compared this kind of self-righteous anger to a hot coal that we pick up to throw at someone else, only to be burned ourself. In George's case, his anger was also burning the rest of his family, who were eager to welcome Rachel back, even if they didn't agree with her choice of mate. For seven weeks of the Mind/Body program, George meditated. For seven weeks, he observed the flow of his thoughts, what occupied his mind. Rachel, Rachel, Rachel. The very thing he wanted most to cut out of his life was hanging in there most tightly. The message that "what we resist persists" got clearer and clearer. When we got to week eight, the subject of which was forgiveness, George finally said, "I'm ready to forgive because I'm tired of being the prisoner of my own anger."

As with forgiving ourselves, the process of forgiving others begins with the recognition that we are holding onto something and that, despite any other person's role in creating the situation, we are the one responsible for what we do with our hurt. If our peace of mind is dependent on what other people do or do not do, we will never have any peace, particularly when, as is often the case, the person that we are holding the grudge against is dead. Taking responsibility for forgiveness is very powerful because it moves us out of the role of helpless victim that fuels our continued anger.

The steps in forgiving others parallel those of forgiving ourselves:

1. Recognizing that we are responsible for what we are holding onto.
2. Confessing our story to ourselves, another person, and God.
3. Looking for the good points in ourself and the other person.
4. Considering whether any specific action needs to be taken.
5. Looking to God for help.
6. Reflecting on what we have learned.

Step One: Taking Responsibility for What We Are Holding Onto

As long as George insisted on blaming Rachel for what she'd done, he couldn't take responsibility for his part of the drama. If it is all the other person's fault, then we stay stuck in our self-righteous pride and can't move toward forgiveness. The position of being one-up means that the other person has to be one-down, and there is no way to forgive one another except as equals. We may not care for the other person's behavior, but condemning them as a person is the way we hold onto blame and block the road to forgiveness. Nathan's statement, "I'm ready to forgive because I'm tired of being the prisoner of my own anger," was taking responsibility for his own role in things—it had nothing to do with what Rachel did or didn't do. It was between Nathan and himself.

Step Two: Confessing Our Story

Part of any healing is being listened to by a neutral party who will not judge. In the heat of our rage, indignation, and hurt, neutrality is not what we are usually looking for. We are more likely to look for support in staying angry. Naturally, it is very easy to find people who will identify with our rage over being victimized. This is a great disservice. We need someone to listen to us without agreeing or disagreeing, which creates the space for us to see things as they are. Some of us are fortunate in having wise friends who can be neutral listeners. Others of us may know wise clergy. Often the neutral listener is a psychotherapist whom we have consulted when, as with George, the pain has become too much to bear. Seeking therapy in such situations, by the way, is never a sign of weakness. It is a sign of strength.

Step Three: Looking for the Good Points

Sometimes in telling our story to a neutral observer, we see things about ourselves that were hidden before. In George's case, he saw his rigidity, his anger, and his self-righteousness which, after some reflection, he decided had probably played a part in Rachel's distance from him as she was growing up. Sometimes, when this happens, we experience a strange reversal. Instead of blaming the other person, we begin to blame ourself instead, which is no better. The way to move through both types of blame is to look for the good points in both parties. With a little help, George could appreciate the good aspects of his fathering and remember the love he felt for Rachel. And in remembering Rachel's good points, her father began to feel how much he missed her.

Step Four: Considering What Actions Need to Be Taken

Sometimes forgiveness is largely a mental and spiritual event, but at other times specific actions are required. In George's case, he needed to talk to his child and make peace. Although there was the possibility that Rachel would reject his overtures out of her own hurt, nonetheless George could be responsible only for his own actions. If she rebuffed him, then forgiveness would have to start anew from that event.

Whenever forgiveness requires that we communicate to the other person our feelings, which usually include anger and hurt, it is imperative to avoid acting out of anger. While expressing feelings is important, it's good counsel to "count to ten first" and calm down a little. If you have gone through steps one to three, it is a good bet that you will be able to communicate with the other person, rather than try to annihilate them. Things said in anger cannot later be retracted and are often very hurtful. They have great potential for escalating the cycle of blame, rather than ending it, because, when we hurt other people out of our anger, we must then go through the process of forgiving ourselves and being forgiven by them. And, make no mistake about it, anger can be a lethal weapon that destroys another person's self-esteem and peace of mind. People are afraid of it for very good reason.

Step Five: Looking to God

Forgiveness is ultimately a gift of grace. We can neither forgive other people nor ourselves entirely out of our own volition. Despite going through all the above steps, our hurt and hatred may still burn on. But what counts most is our desire, our intent, to let it go. If we communicate this desire in heartfelt prayer, we attract grace. Ask God for help in forgiving. Ask to be released from your anger and your hurt.

There's a Buddhist meditation practice called *metta*, or loving-kindness. After feeling loving-kindness toward yourself, you visualize your loved ones and feel loving-kindness toward them. Then you extend the practice to anyone you regard as your enemy. I have found it helpful to imagine such people surrounded by a loving light, and to stay with it until my anger disappears on each occasion. Each time you do it, it gets a little easier to see and send comfort to the wounded child in the other person that was responsible for their lack of judgment.

Step Six: What Have I Learned?

Anthropologist and author Carlos Casteneda tells a story about how our persecutors can turn out to be our teachers. Don Juan was a man of wisdom, a Mexican *brujo*, who was Casteneda's teacher. When he was young, Don Juan's own spiritual teacher indentured him to work for an abusive, dangerous madman who was the foreman of a ranch. He finally escaped and returned to his teacher, incredulous that the teacher would have placed him in such a terrible situation. But the teacher was firm and clear: He knew what Don Juan needed to learn, and he had put him in exactly the right relationship to learn it! Don Juan was sent back to the "petty tyrant" and told to stay centered, no matter what the foreman did to provoke him. After a few years of this, Don Juan had indeed learned the warrior's skill of patience and the ability to keep his center, no matter what the provocation.

Not all of us need to learn Don Juan's lesson of patience. For some of us, the same petty tyrant would be a good teacher of assertiveness who forced us to become more adept at leaving abusive relationships. Or perhaps we would discover a hidden talent for healing that would transform our miserable oppressor into a kindly helpmate. Forgiveness doesn't mean that we have to like our petty tyrants, by the way, although we can certainly learn to appreciate their good points. Forgiveness happens when we can let go of our grudges by learning something and practicing compassion. Then we will no longer need that relationship or others like it as teachers. With this perspective, we can carry on the process of forgiveness with the trust and faith that God—no less than Don Juan's mentor—provides just the right opportunities for our growth.

SELF-ACCEPTANCE, PRIDE, AND HUMILITY

Learning to forgive ourselves and others is evidence of important changes that have occurred in the structure of our personality and thought patterns. One of the most important of these is the development of self-esteem. People sometimes get confused about self-esteem, mistaking it for pride and egotism. Conversely, it's easy to mistake humility for the fearful "let's not rock the boat" mentality of unhealthy guilt, in which we tell ourselves or someone else that they are forgiven while we're still secretly holding onto blame.

Myrin and I once had a Christian spiritual teacher who helped us understand humility through a conversation with a slightly retarded member of our congregation named Mike. At a class one day, Mike was complaining that he wasn't too bright, certainly not as smart as the rest of us. The priest turned on him with surprising force and said, "You certainly are full of yourself!" We were all a bit shocked, since it seemed that Mike's problem was just the opposite.

Then, looking at Mike with a lot of love, he explained that the body of the universe is like the human body, and that we're all different cells and organs in it. "If all your organs wanted to be eyes, Mike, your body would be in trouble. After all, your eyes wouldn't be able to see without the help of your heart. And where would you be without arms and legs, ears and a nose? Who's to say that it's better to be an eye than a liver? So when you complain about not being smart, you are turning down your own unique, God-given place in the scheme of things, and that's downright egotistical!" Mike never complained about not being smart enough again.

The philosopher Martin Buber reminds us that "uniqueness is the essential good of man that is given to him to unfold." When we understand this, we have attained humility. When we don't, we're in Mike's position. Buber once wrote that, "Haughtiness means to contrast oneself with others. The haughty man is not he who knows himself, but he who compares himself with others." Forgiveness—finding the unique good in ourselves and others and letting go of judgment and comparison—is actually a component of humility. Buber says of the humble man:

> Since no one is to him "the other," he knows from within that none lacks some hidden value; knows that there "is no man who does not have his hour." For him, the colours of the world do not blend with one another, rather each soul stands before him in the majesty of its particular existence. In each man there is a priceless treasure that is in no other. Therefore, one shall honour each man for the hidden value that only he and none of his comrades has.
>
> —*The Legend of the Baal-Shem* [p. 45]

FORGIVENESS AS AN ATTITUDE OF NONJUDGMENTALNESS

Buber is talking about humility in much the same way that Campbell talks of the Grail—a state of consciousness in which judgment is suspended and life is seen once again as a Unity rather than defined by the pairs of opposites. In this state of consciousness, where the connection to the greater Source of being is remembered, one knows that no man is "the other." How then can one help being compassionate, suffering with, the other? At the spiritual level, one *is* the other. Jesus spoke of this in the New Testament when he said that whatever we do for the least of our brethren, we do also for him. He was speaking of the Unity that exists beyond the phenomenal world of space and time where things appear separate, defined by the pairs of opposites.

People who have had near-death experiences, temporarily leaving the phenomenal world of time and opposites, are amazed at the state of Unity, which they often describe as a sense of connectedness to all things. In *The Light Beyond*, Raymond Moody, M.D., cites the first-person account of how this experience affected a "hard-driving, no nonsense" businessman following a cardiac arrest:

> The first thing I saw when I awoke in the hospital was a flower, and I cried. Believe it or not, I had never really seen a flower until I came back from death. One big thing I learned when I died was that we are all part of one big, living universe. If we think we can hurt another person or another living thing without hurting ourselves, we are sadly mistaken. I look at a forest or a flower or a bird now, and say, "That is me, part of me." We are connected with all things and if we send love along those connections, then we are happy [p. 34].

The happiness we are seeking, the ability to send love along those connections, is compassion. Another way to think about compassion is as the suspension of judgment. When we size up another person and determine whether we are one-up or one-down, we are judging both of us. If we feel happy about our superiority this time, we will feel bad about our inferiority another time. Judgment cannot lead to lasting happiness. Jesus referred to this when he said in the seventh chapter of the Gospel of Matthew, "Judge not lest you be judged. For with what judgment you judge you shall be judged, and with what measure you mete, it shall be measured to you again." He reminded us to pull out the motes from our own eyes, not to judge the motes in other eyes. In following this advice, we become compassionate and hence happy. We transcend what Eastern philosophy calls the attachment to praise and blame.

The suspension of judgment, as we have already alluded to, in no way implies the suspension of discrimination. These are completely different functions. For example, in forgiving a murderer by being compassionate and understanding the roots of his action in his own pain, we don't let him out of jail until he is hopefully rehabilitated. In forgiving a divorced spouse who battered us, we are not required to marry him again. In forgiving a friend who hurt our feelings, we are required not to overlook her action but to communicate about it.

In *The Power of Myth*, Joseph Campbell tells Wolfram's charming story of how the Grail was brought to earth. While God and the good angels were fighting Satan and the bad angels, the neutral angels brought down the Grail right through the middle of the fray, between the pairs of opposites that create judgment and strife. Whether we speak of Buddha's middle way and his ideal of perfect loving-kindness or the Christian ideal of *agape*, the love one can extend even to an enemy, we are talking about forgiveness. Compassion in action.

St. Francis of Assisi, whose legendary gentleness drew wild animals to play at his feet, left a magnificent statement of compassion in his well-loved prayer:

Lord, make me an instrument of Thy peace.
Where there is hatred let me sow love.
Where there is injury let me sow pardon.
Where there is doubt let me spread faith.
Where there is despair let me bring hope.
Where there is darkness let me bring light.
Where there is sadness let me bring joy.
Grant that I may not so much seek to be consoled as to console,
to be understood as to understand,
to be loved as to love.
For it is in giving that we receive,
And in pardoning that we are pardoned.

SUGGESTIONS FOR THE READER

1. Are you holding onto anything that you haven't forgiven yourself for doing?

2. Are you still the prisoner of someone you have not forgiven? Perhaps there is someone who, until this very moment, you had not even contemplated being able to forgive. Do you think you could bring yourself to begin? If you cannot, then you will remain in the position of victim, a position in which healing from unhealthy guilt cannot occur. It is not worth being a victim.

3. In the resources section at the end of the book, you will find a guided meditation on forgiveness that you might like to try.

CHAPTER NINE

Relationships

The memory of meeting Myrin at an anatomy convention (yes, that's really true) is still vivid. The chemistry was immediate—it was literally love at first sight. We talked until two in the morning the evening that we met, finally leaving the hotel to walk hand-in-hand in the magic of an early spring night. Lost in time, peculiarly close to the majesty of the stars, we stopped at a fountain that seemed as romantic as any in Rome. Sitting silently on its smooth granite wall, we gazed endlessly into each other's eyes. Though tired and bedraggled, neither of us worried about how we looked or whether our mouthwash had worn off. We were lost in the overwhelming sweetness of love's blindness where we see our beloved as perfect, exactly as they are. Suddenly, it's like a state of grace has descended and we are able to see the God in each other.

Psychologists have compared this sudden altered state of consciousness to psychosis. Our reality testing goes on the blink. Obstacles seem to evaporate and everything is possible. We become hopelessly, irrationally optimistic, feeling at one with each other and a larger sense of wholeness. The two lovers inhabit a world of their own, seriously disconnected from everyday reality. My father warned me about this manic, crazy state quite often as I entered my teenage years. "Don't make rash decisions if you happen to fall in love," he would say. "It's like trying to make a decision about buying stocks after drinking a bottle of champagne. You'll live to regret it."

When I fell in love with Myrin, all those reasonable warnings fell on deaf ears, but fortunately everything worked out all right! The experience had a "larger than life" quality to it. In the moment of falling in love, it was as if the reason for living had suddenly been revealed and two halves had become whole. That night by the fountain was an experience outside of time as we usually experience it, a long-awaited reunion across unknowable eons of eternity. Spiritually, falling in love has been compared to the reunion with the lifeforce, the completion of the hero's journey, the mystical union of bride and bridegroom.

LOVE'S PROMISE— A PREVIEW OF COMING ATTRACTIONS

I like to think of this wondrous, but necessarily transient, state of falling in love as a preview of coming attractions, as love's promise of things to come. Like a flash of grace, we are given a vision of what can eventually manifest in a relationship as the partners tread the long path of self-discovery together. But, if we view the preview's inevitable fading away as a "falling out of love," we'll never get the experience of sitting through a whole relationship movie, with its joys and sorrows, its loyalties and betrayals, its anguishes and exultations that make relationship a spiritual path.

Judith Viorst writes, "Infatuation is when you think he's as gorgeous as Robert Redford, as pure as Solzhenitsyn, as funny as Woody Allen, as athletic as Jimmy Connors, and as smart as Albert Einstein. Love is when you realize that he's as gorgeous as Woody Allen, as smart as Jimmy Connors, as funny as Solzhenitsyn, as athletic as Albert Einstein, and nothing like Robert Redford in any category—but you'll take him anyway." Humorous though this may be, it's also the very crux of relationship. Allowing the other person to be who they are, and loving them as they are. And, naturally, how can we do this for another until we can do it for ourself? Relationships are an ongoing course in love and forgiveness. Many mystics, in fact, dissuaded their disciples from leading monastic lives, telling them that marriage and life as a householder was a more difficult but quicker path to Self-realization than monastic celibacy!

Myrin and I were fortunate in understanding that love's initial promise was up to us to fulfill, but that didn't prevent many years of struggling, pain, and confusion—it just gave us the courage to endure! Marriage, a word I'll use generically to apply to any committed relationship or union, is hard, exacting work. If you think otherwise, it's foolhardy to enter one. Our loved ones are like mirrors for us, because in seeing how they react to what we put out, we see ourselves for who we are—our light as well as our shadow. The ideal of relationship is that we will love and support one another in completing the process of growing up, facing our dragons and celebrating the uniqueness that we alone bring into this world.

Pierre Teilhard de Chardin was a paleontologist, poet, philosopher, and priest whose writings embody creation spirituality and the Via Positiva or way of joy. He had a lot to say about relationships with our Self, one another, and the Divine Source of love, which he regarded as an outpouring of blessing. To Teilhard de Chardin, love was a sacred reserve of energy which he deemed the "blood of spiritual evolution." His assertion that we can attain each other only by consummating a union with the Universe points to the mystery of human relationship as a crucible for the Divine alchemy.

Love's promise is that if we are willing to see our relationships as teachers, rather than discard or demean them if they disappoint us, they will lead us to become more self-aware, forgiving and capable of making choices that create happiness and peace of mind. The more we choose to let go of judgments, the more we can relate to the Self in ourselves and others rather than to the ego and its fears. The Sanskrit word *Namasté* is the fulfillment of love's promise. It is a greeting which means *I honor the Universe which dwells within you as peace, love and wisdom*. When we relate to each other's uniqueness with that understanding, we participate in the Divine alchemy where two become One. This is the Via Positiva, the blood of spiritual evolution.

I AM WHO I AM. YOU ARE WHO YOU ARE

I remember a conversation that took place very early one Saturday morning in college as a group of us tumbled through the dorm doors bleary-eyed, just before the 2:00 A.M. curfew. My friend Jeannie had just returned from a date with Bill, her boyfriend of the last several months. He had the basic ingredients she was after. He was intelligent, sensitive, kind, and very good-looking. A little wimpy, though, and not quite as assertive as Jeannie would have liked. He was also what we called a finky dresser. It was definitely not cool to wear gray wool trousers to class in 1965. Blue jeans were the uniform of the day. Jeannie, as usual, was fantasizing about the "great make-over" that would perfect Bill. She would glowingly report how sexy he'd looked in the jeans she had insisted he buy and wear to the jazz club where they'd gone that night. Not surprisingly, Bill got fed up with Jeannie's constant efforts at remaking him in her image, and he moved on to another relationship.

Forgiveness is not just the willingness to work out the hurts that we knowingly or unknowingly inflict on each other. It's also learning to let one another be ourselves—as Rilke says so beautifully, to "succeed in loving the distance between us which enables each to see the other whole against the sky." This requires going beyond the narcissism of thinking that our own way of seeing things is the "right" way. Since we are each the product of specific life experiences, everyone sees the world a little differently, and relationship is an opportunity to appreciate those differences and learn from one another. Although in marriage "two are made as one," we can't reach unity until both parties have grown up, finished the childhood task of separating from their parents, and declared their independence to be themselves. The ideal is not to lose oneself in the other, but to find oneself by helping each other to complete the work of separation that is started, but usually not finished, in childhood.

When Myrin and I were married, the service called for us to exchange red roses with the vow, "I set you free to follow the God within." Then we shared a cup of the water of life. The ceremony was deeply moving, and, although we had no idea of how we would set one another free, it reinforced our sense of spiritual commitment. It was a touchstone to which we could return during the years of growing up together and a promise of things to come.

At first, we figured that the turbulent waters of married life had to do with adjusting to each other's peculiarities. This meant lots of compromises. But it turned out that compromise usually meant a reduction in conflict to tolerable levels where neither of us was miserable but no one was happy either. Yet the original meaning of "compromise" is a far cry from lukewarm adequacy. It comes from the Latin *com*, meaning with or together. The word "promise," in turn, derives from the Latin root *pro* (in behalf of) and *mis* (to give). To compromise is to give each other something for the mutual benefit of both. It is a way of building bridges between different worldviews that allow communication and enrichment, while preserving the integrity of both partners. Before we learn to build bridges, though, we need to understand where the distances are and how we are different.

WHO'S TO BLAME?

In learning to appreciate our differences and set one another free to become who we are, we will recapitulate all the childhood pain that blocks the ability to give and receive love. The less aware the partners are of the frightened child that, to one extent or another, is still alive within us all, the more they will replay the childhood hurt of conditional love and fall into a blame game where finding out "whose fault" this or that is becomes the most frequent shared pastime. The resulting anger and defensiveness tie up a lot of energy that could be used more happily for other purposes. The more the partners begin to see the frightened child in one another—and make the critical shift of supporting its growth rather than blaming the partner for not being fully grown up yet—the more freely love flows, the more creative the partners can be in their daily lives, and the more joyful and alive the family situation becomes.

An important part of helping one another to grow up and separate from the parents we're still carrying around inside ourselves is learning to separate from each other. We learn to do this by locking horns in conflict often enough to begin ferreting out how our old baggage is continuing to weigh down a new relationship. In working through these repetitive conflicts, we begin to see our shadows more clearly. There's an old Zen story, one that I love to tell and retell, that makes this point very well. It concerns an interesting "couple," two monks who were walking in silence by a river at sunrise, early in the spring.

Swollen with the melting snows, the river had overflowed its banks and swamped the small footbridge that was the only point of crossing for many miles. A young woman, in much distress, stood forlornly by the swiftly running river, pleading with her eyes for the monks' help. Sweeping her into his arms, the older monk bore her aloft through the swirling current and put her down safely on the other side. The two monks walked in silence until sunset, when the vows of their order allowed them to talk. The younger monk then turned on his brother with unbridled fury. "How could you have picked that woman up!" he accused. His face grew red as he shook his fists at the older monk. "You, of all people, know the vows of our order. It is forbidden even to think of a woman, let alone to touch one! You have defiled yourself. Indeed, you have shamed the entire order!"

The elder monk turned to him complacently. "My brother," he said. His eyes were soft with the wisdom of forgiveness. "I put that woman down on the other side of the river this morning. It is you who have been carrying her around all day." It's a good bet that the young monk's fury and inability to let go of his anger had more to do with his own unresolved feelings about women than they did with the older monk's actions. He was projecting his own shadow onto his brother's motives. But the wise old monk was too clever to take in the younger monk's shadow projections—in other words, to borrow his guilt and assume blame for something that was not his responsibility.

THE STORY OF DAVID AND SANDY

Distinguishing whose guilt is whose is often neither easy nor clear-cut, especially within the tangled web of a long-term relationship. Consider the case of David and Sandy, whose misappropriation of guilt, childhood fear, and insecurity nearly cost them their marriage. David, though a successful surgeon, was insecure beneath the veneer of all his accomplishments. His way of camouflaging that insecurity was under a self-righteous, know-it-all attitude. A heart surgeon, David often chided Sandy, who was a health-minded and conscientious cook, for putting too much butter on the vegetables. She should, after all, know better and care more for the health of the family. He had other comments about Sandy's part-time nursing career and how she handled the children. Around David, the most casual conversations often turned into long-winded, blaming lectures.

Almost completely out of touch with the fears and insecurities of the frightened child within him, David, like the young monk, projected his emotions onto his wife. David actually thought he was doing Sandy a favor in finding these unfortunate tendencies in her! But, unlike the older monk in the story, Sandy was a great sponge and absorbed David's shadow without question, shouldering the blame that wasn't hers to take because this is what she'd done in her own childhood. Unable to hold her own against David's arrogance, Sandy conformed outwardly to his wishes, all the while feeling angrier and angrier inside, unloved and unappreciated for who she was. Then, when her feelings came out as anger or anxiety, David condemned her "overemotionality," once again cutting off the possibility of communication.

In spite of the distance that grew between them, David put up a good front about the marriage, encouraged by the fact that he believed his own rationalizations. He projected the image of "the perfect couple" and the "perfect parents," and he believed it, using his busy life as a shield from the messages that something was wrong. But Sandy, feeling alone and unloved, was getting progressively more desperate. After ten years of alienation, Sandy met an attractive man at a continuing education course who seemed to value and care for her. He respected her opinions and listened to her feelings. After a friendship of several months, they had a brief affair. But Sandy was quickly overwhelmed with remorse. She began to have anxiety attacks and to wake up at night hyperventilating. She developed headaches, and her childhood asthma recurred.

Unable to contain the guilt any longer, Sandy confessed the affair. David was shattered, and his well-masked insecurity erupted as the angry need to punish her in order to regain control. Hurt and furious, he hurled thunderbolts at her integrity, told her that her behavior was unforgivable, and questioned her ability to mother their children. Fortunately, their intense mutual pain drove them to therapy, where they sorted their guilt and blame into "his," "hers," and "theirs." In therapy, Sandy compared their marriage to a shiny red apple—perfect on the outside, but rotten at the core.

The healing finally began when they stopped blaming one another for Sandy's affair and took mutual responsibility for the events that led up to it. Before we trace the steps of forgiveness through which David and Sandy healed their relationship, grew up, and learned to become themselves, we need to take a closer look at how men and women differ in their basic outlook on the world. Unless these differences are appreciated, it's easy to fall back into blaming one another for our differences instead of deriving strength through our complementarities.

THE MALE AND FEMALE ASPECTS

While men and women are anatomically distinct, their psychological differences are less discrete. According to Carl Jung, man is not all man and woman is not all woman. We each have both masculine and feminine aspects. *The female aspect* is represented by Eros, the relational, connecting "touchy-feely" sense of empathy that is receptive, vulnerable, intuitive, expansive, and retentive. *The male aspect* is represented by Logos, the rational, discriminating, thinking quality of mind that is dominant, protective, and aggressive.

It was easy to see the female aspect in Sandy, who had great people skills, a finely honed sixth sense, and a generosity as big as all outdoors. Sandy, in fact, was generous to a fault, as are many of her colleagues in the nursing profession. Unable to sort out her needs from those of other people, she often gave until she was exhausted, completely unable to say no and carve out any space for herself.

David, on the other hand, had a strong male aspect that wasn't adequately counterbalanced by his female side. He was extremely logical and rational, skills that helped him professionally, but his people skills were rudimentary at best. He often belittled Sandy and their children for being emotional, assuming that they should be logical just the way he was. David's arrogant, know-it-all attitude also made it hard for people to warm up to him because he was a poor listener. David didn't wait for his patients to tell him how they felt, he told them how they *should* feel instead! So, while Sandy found herself too enmeshed in other people's feelings, David could barely engage at all. They were extremes.

The extremes—pure Eros or pure Logos—react to the insecurity on which guilt is based in very different ways. The female aspect is naturally submissive and ruminative, unconcerned with its place in the pecking order. When challenged, Eros retreats from the aggressor and becomes submissive. Biologically, this is a good survival strategy because attackers usually back off from stationary targets. It's hard for a person like Sandy, with a poorly developed male aspect, to be assertive when challenged, so she naturally knuckled under when confronted by David.

The male aspect, on the other hand, is naturally aggressive and active. It instinctually understands that fear and insecurity are like the smell of blood to the pack—they invite attack. Consequently, the male aspect deals with insecurity by building strong defenses against any show of vulnerability. Insecurity shows up not as helplessness, as it did for Sandy, but as an arrogant, cocksure attitude like David's.

I chose the story of David and Sandy not because they are typical but because they are extremes of how males and females cope with insecurity. Each of us has a different mix of male and female aspects that, along with our personal history and the pressures of the society in which we develop, affect our coping styles. Men whose female aspect is particularly well developed are more likely to act like the vulnerable Sandy than the arrogant David. Conversely, insecure women whose male aspect is particularly well developed are more likely to be arrogant and self-righteous like David, rather than guiltily self-effacing like Sandy.

Stop for a moment *and think about yourself. Which is dominant in you, the male or the female aspect? Think about your closest relationship, whether a friendship or a marriage. Which aspect is dominant in the other person?*

If you're not sure, think about how each of you deals with anger. People who are petrified by other people's anger, and who feel worthless and endangered under attack, are more likely to have a dominant female aspect. Those who feel energized by anger, or are at least not terrified by it, more often have a dominant male aspect. As with most dichotomies, black and white is an illusion. Remember that each of us has both aspects. We're talking about degrees here, not the presence or absence of masculine or feminine traits.

GROWING UP TOGETHER

Even though Sandy and David were extreme personality types whose marriage had become painful and stuck, they still had enough of a bond to stay together rather than opt for divorce. Like many couples in trouble, although terribly angry with one another they still felt the underlying love. They could remember the vitality of love's original promise, when for a time they had seen and related to the Self in each other rather than playing out their childhood insecurities. The flame of love, though hidden beneath ten years of hurt, had not been extinguished. It gave them the strength to begin the hard work of helping one another to grow up. This is the process they went through:

Step One: Admitting the Problem

No one can heal a problem they don't think they have. For years Sandy and David lived a myth. They pretended that their relationship was terrific. She turned the other cheek to David's digs and criticisms, keeping up the front like a good martyr. He portrayed their marriage as the pinnacle of perfection and escaped from his feelings through workaholism, an addiction that Sandy actively encouraged because it also protected her from some of her own pain. They continued in this way for over a decade until Sandy's anger finally surfaced in the affair that ended their mutual denial and forced them to admit there was a problem. When David's anger at Sandy was met full force by her own anger for years of "being patronized, ignored, and devalued," they understood very quickly that the affair was just the tip of the iceberg.

Step Two: Getting Through the Blame

The first and most painful phase of David and Sandy's therapy was a rerun of all the blame stored up in their entire marriage. David's fury over her betrayal brought up dozens of past issues and day-to-day grievances—how she left the laundry piled up where it bothered him or refused to stop buttering the vegetables—in short, all the "little," indirect ways that Sandy tried to assert herself instead of confronting David outright. In turn, Sandy's feelings of being "unseen, unknown, and unloved" exploded with a vehemence and rage that surprised them both.

She was harboring grudges from the first year of the marriage, and most of them boiled down to "David's never letting me be myself." David later compared the weeks of trotting out past hurts to lancing a boil. It was most unpleasant, but it drained the poison out. After all, how can we let go of something before we've communicated it or begin to forgive until our grievances have been heard and acknowledged? For Sandy, David's simple apology, "I'm sorry. I never realized how you felt," took a big weight off her heart. She was then able to apologize sincerely for the affair, knowing that he understood what had driven her to it.

Step Three: Finding and Comforting the Wounded Child in One Another

Taking responsibility for our behaviors involves asking questions. Why did Sandy have an affair? The voice of blame says things like, because she's a betrayer, a bad person, immature, stupid, nasty, or malicious. These are value judgments, not reasons. Can you see the difference? Value judgments cut off communication, prevent seeing and learning from the problem, and stand in the way of forgiveness. Asking why goes beyond the blame to the person's own hurt, for what hurtful action doesn't spring in some way from our own pain?

Sandy had an affair because she felt uncared for. In understanding why she had allowed these feelings to go on without asserting herself, Sandy had to go back and discover the frightened child within. Doing some inner child work, Sandy examined her past. Her mother had died when she was just twelve years old, and she grew up an overly responsible child, always protecting her father from his grief and loneliness at the price of denying her own feelings. No wonder she unconsciously repeated the same pattern with David! Then there was the big question of why David often behaved so judgmentally. In combing back through his childhood, David was shocked to realize how angry he felt at the father that he had idealized and tried so hard to please all his life.

Slowly, through therapy and by taking a closer look at their conflicts, Sandy and David learned things about each other and themselves that they hadn't known before. They reached a major turning point when they could see how their fights and disagreements were extensions of their childhood pain. This was the 51 percent point when grace suddenly tipped the balance and blame gave way to compassion. They really wanted to help and comfort each other, not to blame each other and repeat the original wounds. This is what loving relationships are all about. When we can help bring out the best in one another, rather than pointing out the worst, love becomes a vital force that transforms both people and leads to a sure healing of the wounded child.

Step Four: Building Bridges

In addition to their childhood conditioning, David and Sandy also had to build bridges between the extremes of the male and female aspects that they represented. When Sandy felt anxiety, depression, or any strong emotion and reached out to David for support, his old behavior was to withdraw or to criticize. Sandy would then retreat in a dark, angry sulk. When it came to the relational, empathetic world of feelings—the female aspect—David was like a fish out of water. Emotions were alien territory to him, dominated as he was by a logical, rational male aspect. He wasn't trying to be mean or unsupportive; he truly didn't understand how he could help. So when he tried to make Sandy feel better in the only way he knew, by reasoning things out or pointing out why she didn't need to feel how she did, both of them wound up frustrated.

Sandy, whose female aspect was well developed, expected David to be as empathetic as she was. When he didn't pick up on signals because they were literally invisible to him, she concluded that he didn't care. It had never occurred to her—or to him—that they sensed the world in two very different ways. It was as if one person saw in blue and the other in red. Because they hadn't seen their differences clearly before and didn't understand what the problem was, Sandy and David couldn't communicate about feelings. Understanding their problem put an entirely new and blame-free perspective on their relationship, one that created an interesting challenge—building bridges of communication rather than holding angry grudges.

Sandy learned to say things like, "When you withdraw from me and get quiet, it makes me feel even more anxious." David was able to acknowledge her feelings, even though he couldn't understand them, and respond with answers like, "I'm sorry. I know it's hard for you when I do that, but your anxiety makes me uncomfortable. I don't know what to say or how I can help." When Sandy told him that he didn't have to solve her anxiety and that holding her for a few minutes was all she really needed, David was amazed and relieved. Since his male aspect saw the world as a series of equations that all had solutions, he had tended to feel disempowered when he couldn't come up with one.

Sandy taught David that feelings don't need solutions—they just need acknowledgment. David, in turn, shared his male aspect with Sandy and taught her how to keep track of her boundaries: who did or didn't get to enter her emotional space and share her energy. The phone rang one evening while Sandy was cooking. It was a colleague who wanted help with a nursing question that took Sandy fifteen minutes to explain. She hung up the phone angry about the interruption, helpless as usual to define the boundaries between her and the rest of the world. David gave her very clear instructions: "Find out what the person wants, and then stop and think. It's your choice. Just because someone calls doesn't mean you have to drop everything. Do you want to talk to them? If so, when do you want to talk to them? Tell them if and when they can call back."

As simple as this sounds, it took a lot of coaching and practice for Sandy to learn male skills that didn't come naturally. But after several months it became second nature. Likewise, David's attempts to relate to feelings were at first halting, but with time became progressively more natural. Sandy and David learned to enrich one another through their differences, to cherish the distance between them so necessary for them to function as a whole, and to help one another grow up and express the unique potential that each one had to share.

GIVING AND RECEIVING

There's a beautiful little song that goes:

From thee I receive
To thee I give
Together we share
That we both may live.

Giving and receiving are the two acts on which loving relationships are built. We do both many times each day. When the exchange goes smoothly, we feel supported, loving and loved. When it doesn't, we feel anger, frustration, and guilt. Have you ever tried to give something to someone, only to have them reject your offering? Or been afraid to ask, for fear that your request would be rejected? Giving and receiving are the two poles between which the current of love flows, and learning to be honest about what we want to receive, and what we can and cannot give are critical to relationship.

I have a poignant childhood memory from the 1950s, when little girls practiced twirling batons for hours. One day after I dropped mine, it buckled and bent. I took it to my older brother, Alan, ten years my senior. He grabbed both ends of the hollow, metal tube and tried to bend it back by pressing it across his knees. I was bright-eyed and eager with anticipation. Then, suddenly, the strain on the thin metal was too much, and the baton snapped in half.

Alan felt terrible. He took me in his arms and apologized for breaking it, promising that he would buy me another one right away. I was overcome with empathy for him, thinking about how bad he felt. I felt awful that he would spend his money on my baton and go without something for himself, so I started to cry. Not understanding that I was crying tears of empathy, Alan called me a spoiled brat since, after all, he was going to replace the baton. He stomped off in a huff. Despite the tremendous love we had for each other, a miscommunication still got in the way of a very simple act of giving and receiving. If even the pure and uncomplicated love between a sister and brother can get derailed, think about how much harder the act of giving and receiving becomes in more complicated relationships.

The basic problems in giving and receiving are not getting what you want and getting what you don't want!

Not Getting What You Want

Many women who have been socialized to be the "givers" in our society have serious problems getting what they want. These problems stem from one very basic error: *They don't think they should have to ask.* After all, shouldn't everyone be empathetic and intuitive if that's how we are? Shouldn't they know how to read our minds and provide us with our heart's desire without our needing to ask? Isn't this what we do for them?

A woman named Cindy came into a mind/body group the day after her birthday. *Mad.* Why? Because her husband hadn't sent flowers. He was supposed to "know" how much she loved flowers, although in the three years of their marriage he had yet to send her any. "What about asking for them," I prodded. "Asking!" Cindy was outraged. "That takes all the romance out of things." Another woman in the group was quick to point out that anger kills the romance off even faster. This mind-reading requirement is such a universal source of trouble in relationship—and flowers are so symbolic of it—that I call this glitch the "You should have sent me flowers" routine.

The cure for anger over not getting what you want is simple. Ask for it directly and clearly. Explain what you're after to your partner's satisfaction. Then ask whether they are willing to honor your request, and, if not, discuss it. After all, we're under no obligation to honor all the requests that people make of us. That would be ridiculous! The important thing is to communicate clearly about what we want and about whether or not the request can be met.

Getting What You Don't Want

I took an exercise class with some women several years ago. Sometimes several of us stayed around to talk when we were done. Sharon came up with an unusual complaint one week. For her birthday the previous week, her husband had bought her a red negligee. We were all green with envy. "What's your problem?" we chorused. "We wish our husbands would send us red negligees." But Sharon had a different point of view. She thought that the gift wasn't a gift at all, but a request for more sex. We asked her if this is what her husband had told her. "Well, no," she said. "We don't talk about those things." Same problem. If you get what you don't want, you have a real opportunity to learn something that isn't being communicated directly. Growth in relationship is built on communication, and the everyday acts of giving and receiving provide grist for the mill. They give us a chance to stop projecting our unmet needs, wants, and fears on our partner and to learn to talk things out.

FULL CIRCLE TO OUR PARENTS

The process of learning about ourselves through relationships, whether or not they endure, inevitably leads us back full circle to our very first relationship—the one we had with our parents. The common tendency to recreate our original relationship leads to a strange paradox. We often choose partners who remind us of the parent who was the most problematic for us. Adult children of alcoholics, for example, have an unconscious radar that frequently leads them to choose alcoholic mates even though the addiction may not yet have developed during courtship. Children who were physically abused are likely to marry abusive mates. If one or both of our parents was critical, we will choose a mate with the same characteristics.

Freud called this unconscious recreation of our childhood traumas the repetition compulsion—we keep repeating the original wound over and over. A more enlightened view is that the Universe has provided us with the perfect relationship to highlight our childhood wounds so that we can overcome them, transforming their pain into the forgiveness that propels us forward in the hero's journey. At some point, all of us need to make peace with our parents, no matter how angry we are at them or how much they may have hurt us. Unless they are crazy and therefore not responsible for their actions, they have just handed down their pain along the line to us. Poor little child to poor little child. They have done the best they could, and wishing that they could have done better is no help to anyone.

When I do forgiveness work with people, the most common "petty tyrants" on people's lists are their parents. We may reside in grown-up bodies, but, as long as the very sound of mother's voice on the other end of the phone pushes our buttons, we are not free, not grown-up and separated, even though we have lived on our own for years. The motivation to work things out with our parents comes in many ways. Both David and Sandy, for instance, began to develop new adult relationships with their parents when, in the course of their own problems, they recognized how tightly they were still bound to their childhood roles. For some of us, this happens when we have our own children, and, much to our shock and horror, we find ourselves treating them in exactly the same way our parents treated us. And, for some of us, it's only the nearness of our death and God's grace that beckons us to complete our childhoods and form a new relationship with our parents.

Julia was thirty-five the summer that her sudden weight loss and stomach pain turned out to be due to a rapidly growing and untreatable stomach cancer that had already spread to the liver. The doctor told her to put her affairs in order; she would be lucky to live until Christmas. A divorcee with two young boys and a lot of very good friends, Julia was in contact with her mother, but they were not close. An only child, she and her dad had been inseparable as she was growing up, a relationship that threatened Julia's mother. The two had spent years as rivals, though neither would admit it, and when her father died during Julia's senior year in college, she and her mother grew emotionally distant, neither one interested in keeping up the pretense of closeness they had maintained for the father's sake, although they kept in touch and visited each other once or twice a year.

Although the news of her daughter's cancer had brought Julia's mother up from Texas to help out after surgery, the visit had been polite and dutiful but superficial. Her mother had offered to stay, but Julia resolutely sent her home, determined to put things in order with the help of her former husband, to leave a collection of letters for her sons to open on each birthday until they turned twenty-one, to tape a library of stories for them, and then to take her leave from this earth just as soon as possible.

Christmas, and the projected moment of Julia's death, came and went. Much to the surprise of the doctors, her condition remained delicate but unchanged. With every month it grew harder for Julia to go on. The grief and the reality of leaving her children had more time to catch up. And as she mourned for the loss of her relationship with her boys, thinking of all the milestones in their lives that she wouldn't be there to share, she began to get in touch with, and to mourn, her relationship with her own mother.

Julia wanted desperately to die, just to have it all over with. "I'm ready to go now, I've made my peace with God, I've provided for the children," she told me, her eyes filled with tears. "By Easter, for certain, I'll have passed on." But winter rolled around to spring, and poignantly she watched the daffodils bloom from the fat bulbs she had planted with her sons the prior fall as a remembrance of her, a symbol of the continuity of life and the everlasting Spirit. As the spring warmed and the days lengthened into summer's lush radiance, Julia's depression began to lift, and she started to get furious. She was angry with God for not following her plan, for not letting her go before the grief became so powerful. And she was angry with her mother. Angrier than she had realized.

Julia and I joked that she was like the Native American Chief in the Dustin Hoffman movie *Little Big Man*. He'd made his peace with the Great Spirit and lay down on a mountaintop to die. Every few hours, he'd open his eyes, look around, and be quite surprised that he was still alive. In the morning he finally got up, brushed himself off and said philosophically, "Well, I guess it wasn't my time, after all." But, in Julia's case, the doctors remained quite sure that it was her time, for while the disease had inexplicably slowed to a snail's pace, she was still dangerously ill. Julia had been meditating since her diagnosis, both to cope with the anxiety and as a spiritual exercise, a way to become closer to God. But suddenly she could barely concentrate. No sooner would she close her eyes than she would be overcome with restlessness and anxiety, and she would give up.

We discussed her problem, and Julia agreed to just stick with her feelings and see where they led her. Pretty soon, she began to have childhood memories of her mother and father. She remembered a time in first or second grade when she'd come home from school all excited about getting a perfect score on her spelling test for the second week in a row. Her father was delighted, but her mother actually accused her of cheating! She was in tears as she recalled the hurt and anger she'd felt when her joy was converted into the need to defend herself. No matter how well she did, how pretty she looked, or how hard she tried, Julia's mother always found some way to tear her down. She was amazed at the rage inside herself, the amount of hurt in the little Julia whose feelings were as vibrant and unresolved at age thirty-six as they had been at seven, eight, and nine.

As soon as the memories welled up, Julia had a strong inner feeling that she couldn't let go and die until she had healed her relationship with her mother, and that only then would her relationship with Matt and Paul, her seven- and nine-year-old sons, be complete. She started the forgiveness process we discussed in the last chapter, and, when she got to the fourth step—considering what action she needed to take—she realized that she had to tell her mother how she felt, whether or not it actually changed the relationship. But she was too scared—that in revealing the depth of her hurt and anger, her mother would somehow push her away and reject her again. So she began the healing mentally, imagining herself back in her childhood home, at first just sitting with her mother silently, and then beginning to talk to her, telling her how scared she was, how much she needed to be loved and accepted. The conversations, though, were one way. She had hoped that her mother would speak, but there was only silence.

It was late fall, a year since the daffodils had been planted, and the fifteenth anniversary of her father's death. Julia was very weak, but her former husband drove her and their sons to the cemetery where her father was buried. They brought a trowel and the same kind of fat daffodil bulbs that they'd planted for Julia the year before. The boys brushed the dried leaves from the gravesite and planted the bulbs, as their mother told them stories of the grandfather they had never known. When the planting was finished, all four of them sat together in silence, and, in the quiet of her heart, Julia asked her father for help in understanding her mother, the woman who had been his wife.

That fall day, fifteen years after his death, Julia reexperienced the safety and peace of her father's love, his love both for her and her mother. And then suddenly she felt the pain, the terror and fright her mother may have felt believing she would lose her husband's love to Julia. Tears began to flow, tears of compassion for the frightened child within her mother who had been so afraid of losing her father's love that she couldn't fully open her heart to her own child. Julia was overwhelmed with love for her mother and compassion for her pain, and she wanted very much for the boys who had never known their grandfather to know their grandmother as she herself had been unable to do.

That night Julia called her mother and took a very big risk. She asked her to fly up and take care of her until she died. At the other end of the phone, her mother began to cry, so touched that the child she had been distant from for so long had welcomed her back into her life. Julia's mother came to care for her daughter and her grandsons during the bittersweet holiday season that marked the final cycle of Julia's growing up. She lived for one more month, until Christmas, grateful for that year of grace during which she and her mother healed and grew up, the year during which the silent and powerful presence of the Third—the One who reconciles in mercy—forgave them both.

This is the story of our growth as human beings and how in our ability to care for one another, to accept one another, and ultimately to love one another, we discover our godhood.

When you find the Light within you
You will know that you have always
Been in the center of wisdom.
As you probe deeper into who you really are
With your lightedness and your confusion
With your angers, longings and distortions
You will find the true living God.
Then you will say
I have known you all my life
and I have called you by many different names.
I have called you mother and father and child

I have called you lover.
I have called you son and flowers.
I have called you my heart.
But I never, until this moment,
called you Myself.

Emmanuel's Book: A Manual for Living Comfortably in the Cosmos
Compiled by Pat Rodegast and Judith Stanton

SUGGESTIONS FOR THE READER

1. Can you identify with the male and female aspects? How do the essential differences affect you and your relationships?

2. Where are you in the process of communications, growing up, and forgiveness within your major relationship? If you need help, are you able to ask for it?

3. Where are you in the process of forgiving your parents?

CHAPTER TEN

Spiritual Exercises and Resources

The psychological and spiritual journey of soul mending is without beginning and without end. Although we may have been unaware of it, our soul has always been seeking for its Source of being. Our problems, mistakes, sufferings, and regrets have been no less a part of our innate movement toward that wholeness than have our conscious efforts to live a life of compassion and love. The journey never ends because our souls continue to grow in wisdom and experience, both in this temporal life and in worlds unseen. We are on a journey with no end and no goal other than living this very moment in its fullness, saying yes to life.

Our ability to say yes, to surrender to the moment—no matter how joyful, sad, loving, or frightening—varies. Sometimes we are in the flow. We can feel the wholeness. At other times, we feel washed adrift by the tides of worry and fear. It doesn't matter. As Joseph Campbell says, the best we can do is intend the good, intend the moment. A monk was once asked what they did up there in the monastery all day. His answer was, "We fall and get up again. Fall and get up again. Fall and get up again." So it is with this life.

When you are up, share your joy. When you are down, share your sorrow. This is all it takes to live the authentic life. If you do this, you will enter into the mystery of compassion, sharing with another. Jesus alluded to this act when he said, "When two or more of you are gathered in my name, there am I in the midst of you." In sharing, we are joined by that Third, as P. L. Travers expresses it, that One who reconciles.

PRACTICES OF REMEMBERING

There are practices that can help us along our journey. They all have one purpose—they help us to remember that the Source of our being is love.

Music is the delight of the soul. It is alive with memories and feelings. Every note that J. S. Bach wrote was dedicated to Christ. You can feel Bach's relationship to the Spirit in his music, and you can share in his ecstasy. There is spiritual music of all kinds. Rock and roll is spiritual when it ignites our impulse to life and awakens our energies. Chanting, devotional music, and the natural sounds of birds and wind, ocean and laughter—these also are spiritual music.

Meditation, in which we leave the world for a little while to enter the Silence of breath or mantra, prepares us to enter into life as a meditation. When we can do this, we recognize that there is no division between the mundane and the holy. Eating a piece of chocolate cake with gratitude and attention to the delight is no less spiritual than prayer. Guided meditations lead us into a particular frame of reference where we can experience familiar things through the wise eye of the Self. You will find three such guided meditations, or inner wisdom exercises, later in the chapter.

Gratitude is a measure of our happiness and a reminder to find our happiness. It keeps us on track. I went to a prayer service once where a priest-healer started with a moment of gratitude for what didn't need healing. When we get lost in what is broken, we can recenter by remembering what is whole—as Rabbi Nachman put it, looking for the good. When out walking, say a silent thank-you for the trees. When you see the face of a loved one, give thanks. As you walk, be grateful for your legs. This is the basis of the Jewish custom of praying frequently throughout the day by thanking God for the little things—a prayer over washing the hands and one for entering the house, a prayer when seeing the first star each night. Gratitude is remembrance.

Prayer is our recognition that God is not wholly other, but part of ourselves. Joseph Campbell points out that the Eastern symbol of yin and yang, the opposites, is a light semicircle with a tail, interdigitating with a dark one. But each has a little eye, a little spot of the other color. Otherwise the two would be wholly other, they could not relate. In prayer, the infinite part of us remembers that it is not wholly other, but part of the infinite consciousness of God. It is good to pray in a way that helps you feel intimate with God, rather than other. Rabbi Nachman suggests that we pray to God as though we were talking to our best friend and to tell Him everything—fears, complaints, hopes, and dreams. God is a good listener.

Selfless service (*seva*) is a spiritual practice recommended in every religion, but one that we must distinguish from the guilty need to rescue. Selfless service comes not from need but from compassion. In *seva*, we really feel the truth of the adage that to give is to receive. I met a lawyer once who spent his vacation in Calcutta helping Mother Teresa and the Sisters of Mercy. While he didn't expect a glamorous vacation, he got a little more than he bargained for. His job was to carry the dead bodies to the burning grounds. It was the best vacation he ever had. But we don't have to go to Calcutta to be of service. We don't even have to leave our own homes. When we see that a loved one has some need, and we act from loving-kindness to fill that need, we are performing *seva*.

Study is a source of wisdom. People who have near-death experiences return not only with the sense that love is the most important thing, but that love awakens the desire for wisdom. They say that love and wisdom are the only two things we take with us from this life, because they are the substance of our souls. I have included at the end of this chapter a resource list of titles that I cited and a few others that have been important to me. A good book is like a living teacher. It talks to you. These days, even if we're on the go, we can be spoken to by books on audiocassette. *A Course in Miracles*, for example, is on audiocassette tape, and you can listen as you drive. *The Power of Myth* is available on videotape, and you can benefit from the presence of a great spiritual teacher in your own home. There are fine audios and videos available from most spiritual groups that are an excellent supplement to reading.

Putting aside time is the spiritual practice that supports all the others. You will not get to the others if there is no time. Perhaps there is an hour in the evening when you can unwind, listen to music, or walk, or meditate, or pray. Even on days when time slips through your fingers, there are the moments in bed, before you fall asleep. The Jewish mystics believe that King David composed all the psalms while meditating in his bed.

TOUCHSTONES FOR REMEMBERING

Touchstones are things that remind us of holy moments. While I was writing this book, my mother was in the last stages of her life. Though a sad time, it was also a wonderful time because we became closer than we had been before. She died while I was working on the revisions to the manuscript. The day and night and morning through which she labored to leave this world and give birth to her soul were among the finest hours of my life. The whole family shared the day and evening with her until late into the night. Then my brother Alan, my son Justin, and I sat through with her until she left her body the next morning. We held her and prayed for her. I sang to her: "Swing Low, Sweet Chariot," Hebrew lullabies, Indian chants, "Amazing Grace," and "Some Enchanted Evening," the song that she and my father fell in love to.

At about 10:00 P.M. she finished saying goodbye to each of us and then told us jokes until she finally fell asleep, waiting for the moment of separation from her body. As we said our goodbyes, Mom and I exchanged gifts. I asked what quality of mine she wanted, and she told me that she admired my compassion. I, in turn, was a great admirer of her courage. Through our eyes and hearts and hands, we made a gift of these qualities to each other's souls.

My mother died on March 18, 1989, the day after Saint Patrick's Day. Her long-time health aide and devoted companion, Olivia, had brought her a yellow rose tinted green for the occasion. It was a fitting parting, since Mom had always joked that she wanted yellow roses at her funeral, as long as they weren't too expensive. They were expensive, but we had dozens of them anyway! I pressed two roses as touchstones, the one that had lain on her pillow all the day and night as she took her leave of this world, and one from her funeral. They remind me of my mother and the indomitability of the human spirit. They remind me of God's grace. But, particularly, they remind me to have courage because I know that I am not alone.

In my meditation space, there are many other touchstones. There is a wooden heart carved out of the crook of an applewood branch that a friend rescued from the fire as the shape of the heart began to appear among the embers. When he had lovingly carved and sanded and polished it, he gave it to me and Myrin for a wedding present since, in the heart, two halves are made a whole. The heart is a touchstone for our love. There are pictures of saints and pictures of a baby. There is a picture of me as a little girl. Special stones that were picked up at holy moments, a piece of rock with raw opal in it given to me by a spiritual teacher, and a rock shaped incredibly like a human breast that reminds me of the gifts of the mother—the Goddess.

Two little plastic geese remind me of our special friend Celia Thaxter

Hubbard, who humorously refers to herself as a channel for Mother Goose. Celia sometimes sends Myrin and me "goose-o-grams" filled with spiritual books, funny things, "goose flashes" of intuition, and sacred items that I often pass along to others. A pair of miniature wooden sandals from the Hindu tradition reminds me of my colleagues and dear friends from the Mind/Body Clinic who gave them to me. They are touchstones for friendship and shared dreams.

I led a workshop on spirituality and daily life at Wellspring, a supportive community for people with cancer in Watertown, Massachusetts. I wanted to begin our day with a sharing, going around the circle from person to person. There is a Native American tradition of passing the talking stick on such occasions and letting the Great Spirit communicate through you. Similarly, I like to pass around a sacred object, a touchstone. I had forgotten the rose crystal heart I had planned to bring, so I turned to the group and asked whether anyone had a touchstone. People reached down their shirts for crystals, medals, and rings hung over their hearts. Purses opened and out came wonderful stones and pieces of ancient pottery. One woman had even brought along a lingam from India, sacred objects that look like smooth, stone eggs found only in one river valley. As we went around the circle, passing around an ancient pottery shard, we shared some of the stories of our touchstones. In that sharing, we helped one another remember the Spirit and the wonderful, often serendipitous ways that it touches us and helps us remember who we really are.

The Native Americans similarly have touchstones for remembering. They carry these items in a deerskin pouch called a medicine bag. Remembering is powerful medicine for healing a soul. What are your touchstones? Try gathering them together in a place that you can use for meditating, journal writing, reading, listening. Create a sacred place for yourself and, when you go there, you can leave the responsibilites of this world behind and remember your connection to a larger sphere of being.

INNER WISDOM EXERCISES (GUIDED MEDITATIONS)

The following guided meditations can help you along the way from guilt to forgiveness. They are meant to help your soul to heal. You can tape them slowly and with love, preferably to a musical background that I will suggest but that you may wish to change. If you prefer, you can order them prerecorded, with me as your guide, as indicated later in the chapter.

Before settling down to tape these exercises, relax. Take a walk or a soak in the tub. Have a good stretch. Then close your eyes and center yourself on your breath. Witness for a few minutes, spend a little time enjoying your inner child, or center yourself with a meditation. Then you will be ready to speak from your heart. As you do, spontaneous changes will occur in the scripts. In fact, every time I use these meditations at a workshop, they come out differently. Go with the inner flow. And enjoy yourself. If, for any reason, these exercises "feel" wrong to you at this time, don't do them.

Healing the Inner Child

I have written this meditation out of my heart. It has been influenced in parts by meditations of Bernie Siegel, Louise Hay, and the thousands of people who have heard it at my workshops, responded to it, and thereby helped it to become alive.

Suggested music:

Pachelbel Canon in D Minor
performed by Daniel Kobialka on the audiotape *Timeless Motion*

—Li-Sem Enterprises, Inc.
1775 Old Country Road, #9
Belmont, CA 94002

Take a deep breath and gently close your eyes. Give a few big sighs . . . sighs of relief . . . and see if your body wants to stretch a little . . . or yawn . . .

Now pay attention to the natural rhythm of your breathing. Feel your body rise gently as you breathe in, and relax as you breathe out . . . (pause for several breaths) . . . every outbreath is an opportunity to let go . . . to relax a little bit more . . . to feel the comfortable heaviness and warmth of your body . . .

And as you relax, you can follow your mind back into the storehouse of special memories . . . back into a very peaceful, magical place from your childhood . . . Your own secret place—just as it was or just as you would have liked it to be . . . (pause). Here, in your nest, you can look out on the world and enjoy the colors . . . the sounds . . . the fragrances . . . and the special feeling of comfort in your own little corner of the world.

And, as you relax, you can find your child-self here . . . Little [name of whoever the recording is for] is here, always here . . . waiting for you . . . for you know [him or her] better and love her more than any other person in the world (pause). Take a good look at her. How old is she? What is she wearing? How does she appear to you? . . .

She is happy to see you, her very best friend . . . Look into her eyes . . . and feel the smile that is growing inside both your hearts. As the closeness grows, go to her. Hug and hold her . . . Feel her joy and her love for you . . . she's been waiting for this for a long time.

It's been so long since she's seen you . . . and there's so much to tell. She may want to tell you in words . . . in pictures . . . or in feelings. This is her *time. All* you *need to do is listen. There's no need to respond just now. Only to listen . . . and be there for her . . . no matter what she has been through, what she may have done, what experiences she has had . . . (long pause).*

When she is done, let her feel your compassion through your eyes and your heart . . . Comfort her . . . Let her know that you will never leave her again . . . that you will always be there for her . . . that, no matter what happens, you will always love her and help her . . . for she has waited all her life to know this . . .

Now let her take you by the hand, and follow her through a sunlit meadow . . . (pause). She wants to show you how beautiful the flowers are . . . and the grasses. She wants to introduce you to the birds and to the wind . . . She wants to take you to a secret place where she has hidden a special gift for you . . . a gift that will help you on your way . . . When you come to that secret place, there is a treasure chest . . . and when she opens it, your gift is inside . . . Take it and thank her. Let her know that you will be back soon . . . That you have never really left . . . Give her a hug and say goodbye for now . . . just for now, because she is always there inside you.

Gradually fade out the music over the next minute as you read the following instructions for reorienting to the room.

. . . And come back to the room whenever you're ready . . . taking your time . . . enjoying the feelings of love and caring, and knowing with complete certainty that you have always *been worthy of love.*

Forgiveness

I have developed this meditation through the years and found it an excellent adjunct to the six-step process of forgiving other people or oneself. Before you go into the meditation, decide who needs forgiveness, but don't be surprised if someone else appears. It is always a good idea to start forgiving the small hurts first, rather than starting this kind of work with your most vibrant enemy.

Suggested music:

Crimson Collection, Volume Five
"Mender of Hearts"
Singh Kaur and Kim Robertson

—Invincible
P.O. Box 13054
Phoenix, AZ 85002

The performers call this music "a love song in the purest sense—a love song to the infinite within each of us and the infinite that unites us all, the one who is the mender of all hearts, the mender of the wounds of life . . . the sustainer of all."

Take a deep breath and gently close your eyes. Give a few big sighs . . . sighs of relief . . . and see if your body wants to stretch a little . . . or yawn . . . (pause).

Now pay attention to the natural rhythm of your breathing. Feel your body rise gently as you breathe in and relax as you breathe out . . . (pause for several breaths) . . . every outbreath is an opportunity to let go . . . to relax a little bit more, to let your body sink down . . . and to feel the comfortable heaviness and warmth . . . (pause).

And you can travel through your mind to the meadows of your innermost being . . . to a sunlit clearing fresh with the mild, fragrant breezes of spring . . . As you breathe, you can relax into the warmth of the sun and feel the wind caress your body and ruffle your clothing . . . you can attune yourself more and more to the delightful sights and sounds and fragrances . . . the grasses, trees, and flowers . . . (pause) . . . the birds and butterflies . . . (pause) . . . the abundance of life in the meadow . . . and the sounds of the crickets and the wind in the trees . . . and you can feel the peace here in this special place . . . and the lifeforce of the awakening spring . . . (pause).

And you can feel the lifeforce in your own body . . . feel it resonating with the meadow . . . feel it as joy . . . (pause) . . . And the meadow is a place of safety, truth, and peace . . . a place of wisdom within yourself where you can always come . . . and within the meadow are many special places you can discover . . . places where you can feel your own power . . . (pause) . . . and places where you can feel especially cozy and safe . . . (pause).

Around the edge of the meadow are openings to different paths—the life experiences you have had . . . paths over spacious, sunlit hills, and through dark, narrow valleys . . . paths through wooded labyrinths and vast open spaces . . . and each of the paths, whether high or low, is like a rainbow . . . for it has a pot of gold . . . a gift of learning . . . at its end.

Nestled in the safety of your own special place, you can look down into the paths of your life experiences . . . at relationships you've had with other people . . . (read in a slightly louder voice) . . . *and choose one where anger, hurt, or guilt or some other emotion still blocks the way to forgiveness . . . (pause) . . . and, in a moment, you will* see *a symbolic image of that emotion walking down the path to meet you at the edge of the meadow . . . to bring you the gift of its teachings . . . (pause).*

Bring your inner emotional messenger to the place of greatest comfort for you in the meadow. It may be a power-place or a safe-place. Since you have changed since you last contacted this feeling, you may want to make your messenger smaller or larger . . .

Settle down and bring the situation that needs forgiveness to mind now . . . (long pause) . . . Ask your emotion how it protected you in that situation . . . (long pause) . . . and thank it for its help . . . Ask it if there are other ways for you to feel safe now—ways that open your heart (long pause) . . . And ask what it has to teach you about the other person . . . (long pause) . . . and about yourself . . . (long pause) . . .

Thank it for its teachings and return the favor by setting it free—letting its energy flow back to the lifesource—as a bird or a flower or a burst of light. Know that it will arise spontaneously wherever needed—free to form and to fade away . . . free to be spontaneously itself.

Feel the lifeforce in the sturdy shoots of new growth all around you . . . Bow in your heart to the author of life . . . to yourself . . . to those who have exchanged love's teachings with you in the form of hurt . . . and know that you are both forgiven . . . now and forever . . .

Begin to fade the music out here for about a minute, and then read the reorientation.

And whenever you feel ready . . . taking your time . . . come back to the room, a little lighter than when you left.

Gratitude and Healing

The body is a great mystery. As a scientist, I used to sit for hours in rapt wonder at its magnificent structure, of the microcosmic worlds within us. When we take time to be grateful for our lives and the very bodies that are our vehicles in this life, we become more respectful of the marvelous creation that we are and help our bodies to relax and heal.

Suggested music:

> *Jesu, Joy of Man's Desiring,* Bach
> performed by Daniel Kobialka on the audiotape *Path of Joy*
>
> —Li-Sem Enterprises
> 1775 Old Country Rd. #9
> Belmont, CA 94002

Take a deep breath and gently close your eyes. Give a few big sighs . . . sighs of relief . . . and see if your body wants to stretch a little . . . or yawn . . . (pause).

Now pay attention to the rhythm of your breathing . . . Feel your body rise gently as you breathe in, and relax as you breathe out . . . (pause for several breaths) . . . every outbreath is an opportunity to let go . . . to feel the pleasant warmth and heaviness of your body . . . a little more on each outbreath . . . (pause).

Now, as you breathe in, imagine your breath as a stream of warm, loving light entering through the top of your head. Let it fill your forehead and eyes . . . your brain . . . your ears . . . and nose . . . feel the light warm and relax your tongue, your jaws, and your throat. Let your whole head float in an ocean of warm light . . . growing brighter and brighter with each breath . . . (pause) . . . Thank your eyes for the miracle of sight . . . your nose for the fragrance of roses and hot coffee on cold mornings (or whatever you like) . . . your eyes for the richness that sound is . . . your tongue for the pleasure of taste . . . and let the light fill and heal every cell of your senses . . .

Breathe the light into your neck . . . let it expand gently into your shoulders . . . and breathe it down your arms . . . and into your hands . . . right to the tips of your fingers . . . Thank your arms and hands for all you have created and touched with your life . . . All the people you have hugged and held to your heart . . . Rest in the warmth and love of the light . . . light that grows brighter with every breath . . .

And breathe the warm light into your lungs and your heart . . . feeling it penetrate your entire chest, filling every organ, every cell with love. As you breathe, send gratitude to your lungs for bringing in the energy of life—and to your heart for sending life to all the cells of your body for serving you so well for all these years . . . rest in the gratitude and love . . . in the light that continues to grow brighter with each breath . . . (pause).

And breathe the light into your belly, feeling it penetrate deeply into your center, into the organs of digestion and reproduction . . . and sense the miracle of your body . . . the mystery of procreation and of the ability to beget life . . . let the light expand through your torso and down into your buttocks . . . growing warmer and brighter . . . balancing and healing all the cells of your body . . .

Breathe the light into your thighs . . . into bone and muscle, nerve and skin, alive with the energy of light . . . comforted in your caring and your love . . . and let the light expand into your calves . . . and your feet . . . right to the soles of your feet . . . feeling gratitude for the gift of walking . . . letting the lovelight grow brighter and brighter . . .

Rest in the fullness of the light . . . enjoying the lifeforce . . . and, if there is any place in your body that needs to relax or to heal, direct the light there and hold that part of yourself with the same love you would give to a hurt child . . . (pause).

Now, as you breathe, sense how the light radiates out from your body . . . just as a light shines in the darkness, surrounding you in a cocoon of love . . . and you can sense that cocoon extending all around your body, above and below you, and to all sides, for about three feet . . . like a giant cocoon . . . a place of complete safety where you can recharge your body and your mind . . . (pause).

And you can imagine the light around other people . . . surrounding them with the same radiance of love, gratitude, and healing . . . see your loved ones in the light . . . see those who you think of as your enemies in the light . . . then let the light expand until you can imagine the entire world as an orb of light . . . (pause) . . . amidst a universe of light (pause) all connected . . . all at peace . . . and feel the wonder and majesty of creation . . . (pause). Now for a minute or two just rest . . . just breathe . . . returning to the warm, comfortable feelings within you . . . (long pause).

Begin fading out the music now, and then read the instructions for reorientation.

And now, begin to reorient yourself to the room . . . slowly and at your own pace . . . bringing the peace and gratitude back with you.

READING LIST

Most of these titles are books that I have mentioned in the text. Others are books that are alive for me and that I hope you will also enjoy. I am grateful to the authors of these books for their wisdom that I have been able to share with you.

Shame and the Inner Child

Beattie, Melody. *Codependent No More.* New York: Harper/Hazelden, 1987.

Berne, Eric, M.D. *Games People Play.* New York: Ballantine Books, 1964.

Bradshaw, John. *Healing the Shame That Binds You.* Deerfield Beach, FL: Health Communications, Inc., 1988.

Kaufman, Gershen. *Shame: The Power of Caring.* Rochester, VT: Schenkman Books, Inc., 1985.

LeBoutillier, Megan. *Little Miss Perfect.* Denver CO: MAC Publishing, 1987.

Miller, Alice. *The Drama of the Gifted Child: The Search for the True Self.* New York: Basic Books, 1981.

Miller, Alice. *For Your Own Good.* New York: Farrar, Straus and Giroux, 1983.

Missildine, W. Hugh, M.D. *Your Inner Child of the Past.* New York: Pocket Books, 1963.

TA: The Total Handbook of Transactional Analysis. Englewood Cliffs, NJ: Prentice Hall, 1979.

Whitfield, Charles L., M.D. *Healing the Child Within.* Deerfield Beach, FL: Health Communications, Inc., 1987.

Wholey, Dennis. *Becoming Your Own Parent.* New York: Doubleday, 1988.

Woititz, Janet, Ed.D. *Adult Children of Alcoholics.* Pompano Beach, FL: Health Communications, Inc., 1983.

Psychology and Mythology

Bly, Robert. *A Little Book on the Human Shadow.* San Francisco: Harper and Row, 1988.

Branden, Nathaniel. *Honoring the Self.* Los Angeles: Jeremy Tarcher, Inc., 1983.

Branden, Nathaniel. *The Psychology of Self-Esteem.* New York: Bantam Books, 1969.

Campbell, Joseph. *Creative Mythology: The Masks of God.* New York: Penguin Books, 1976.

Campbell, Joseph. *The Hero with a Thousand Faces.* Princeton, NJ: Princeton University Press, 1968.

Campbell, Joseph, ed. *The Portable Jung.* New York: Penguin Books, 1971.

Campbell, Joseph, with Bill Moyers. *The Power of Myth.* New York: Doubleday, 1988.

Hardy, Jean. *A Psychology with a Soul: Psychosynthesis in Evolutionary Context.* London: Rutledge and Kegan Paul, Ltd., 1987.

Houston, Jean. *The Search for the Beloved: Journeys in Sacred Psychology.* Los Angeles: Jeremy P. Tarcher, Inc., 1987

Jung, Carl G. *Man and His Symbols.* New York: Doubleday, 1964.

La Berge, Stephen. *Lucid Dreaming.* New York, Ballantine Books, 1985.

Lerner, Harriet Goldhor, Ph.D. *The Dance of Anger: A Woman's Guide to Changing the Patterns of Intimate Relationships.* New York: Harper and Row (Perennial Library), 1986.

Perera, Sylvia Brinton. *The Scapegoat Complex: Toward a Mythology of Shadow and Guilt.* Toronto, Canada: Inner City Books, 1980.

Seifert, Theodor. *Snow White: Life Almost Lost.* Wilmette, IL: Chiron Publications, 1983.

Siegel, Bernie S., M.D. *Peace, Love and Healing.* New York: Harper and Row, 1989.

Tavris, Carol. *Anger: The Misunderstood Emotion.* New York: Touchstone Books, 1982.

Taylor, Jeremy. *Dreamwork: Techniques for Discovering the Creative Power in Dreams.* New York: Paulist Press, 1983.

Wilmer, Harry A., M.D. *Practical Jung.* Wilmette, IL: Chiron Publications, 1987.

Woodman, Marion. *Addiction to Perfection: The Still Unravished Bride.* Toronto, Canada: Inner City Books, 1982.

Near-Death and Other First-Person Experiences

Frankl, Viktor. *Man's Search for Meaning.* New York: Pocket Books, 1959.

An Interrupted Life: The Diaries of Etty Hillesum, 1941–1945. New York: Washington Square Press, 1981.

Lapierre, Dominique. *The City of Joy.* New York: Warner Books, 1985.

Moody, Raymond. *The Light Beyond.* New York: Bantam, 1988.

Ring, Kenneth. *Heading Toward Omega: In Search of the Meaning of the Near-Death Experience.* New York: William Morrow and Co., 1985.

Weiss, Brian L., M.D. *Many Lives, Many Masters.* Fireside Books: New York, 1988.

Philosophy and Religion

Buber, Martin. *The Legend of the Baal-Shem.* New York: Schocken Books, 1969.

A Course in Miracles. Farmingdale, NY: Foundation for Inner Peace, 1975.

Dossey, Larry, M.D. *Recovering the Soul.* New York: Bantam Books, 1989.

Fox, Matthew. *The Coming of the Cosmic Christ.* San Francisco: Harper and Row, 1988.

Fox, Matthew. *Original Blessing: A Primer in Creation Spirituality.* Santa Fe, N.M.: Bear and Co., 1983.

How to Know God: The Yoga Aphorisms of Patanjali. Trans. by Swami Prabhavananda and Christopher Isherwood. New York: New American Library, 1953.

Huxley, Aldous. *The Doors of Perception.* New York: Harper and Row, 1954.

Jacobs, Louis. *Jewish Mystical Testimonies.* New York: Schocken Books, 1977.

James, William. *The Varieties of Religious Experience.* New York: Mentor, 1958.

Jampolsky, Gerald. *Love Is Letting Go of Fear.* Berkeley, CA: Celestial Arts, 1979.

Nachman, Rabbi. *Outpouring of the Soul.* Jerusalem: Breslov Research Institute, 1980.

Nachman, Rabbi. *Restore My Soul.* Jerusalem: Breslov Research Institute, 1980.

Narashima, B. V., Swami. *Self Realization: The Life and Teachings of Sri Ramana Maharshi.* Tiruvannamalai, India: T. N. Venkataraman, 1985.

Pagels, Elaine. *Adam, Eve and the Serpent.* New York: Random House, 1988.

Pagels, Elaine, ed. *The Gnostic Gospels.* New York: Vintage Books, 1981.

Robinson, James M., ed. *The Nag Hammadi Library* (Translations of the Gnostic Scriptures). San Francisco: Harper and Row, 1988.

Rodegast, Pat, and Stanton, Judith, eds. *Emmanuel's Book: A Manual for Living Comfortably in the Cosmos.* New York: Bantam Books, 1985.

Smith, Huston. *The Religions of Man.* New York: Harper and Row, 1958.

The Song of God: Bhagavad-Gita. Trans. by Swami Prabhavananda and Christopher Isherwood. New York: Mentor Books, 1944.

Meditation

Benson, Herbert, and Miriam Z. Klipper. *The Relaxation Response.* New York: Avon Books, 1976.

Borysenko, Joan. *Minding the Body, Mending the Mind.* New York: Bantam Books, 1988.

Gallagher, Blance Marie. *Meditations with Teilhard de Chardin.* Santa Fe, N.M.: Bear and Company, 1988.

Goleman, Daniel. *The Meditative Mind: The Varieties of Meditative Experience.* Los Angeles: Jeremy P. Tarcher, Inc., 1987.

Kaplan, Aryeh. *Jewish Meditation: A Practical Guide.* New York: Schocken Books, 1985.

Kabat-Zinn, Jon. *Full Catastrophe Living.* New York: Delacorte Press, 1990.

Levine, Stephen. *A Gradual Awakening.* New York: Anchor Books, 1979.

Muktananda, Swami. *Meditate.* Albany: State University of New York Press, 1980.

Pennington, Basil M. *Centering Prayer: Renewing an Ancient Christian Prayer Form.* New York: Image Books, 1982.

Thich Nhat Hanh. *Being Peace.* Berkeley, CA: Parallax Press, 1987.

Thich Nhat Hanh. *The Miracle of Mindfulness! A Manual of Meditation.* Boston: Beacon Press, 1976.

ON AUDIOCASSETTE: JOAN'S TAPES

Love Is the Lesson is a seven-tape set consisting of guided meditations, designed to promote inner wisdom and healing.

1. *Breath of Life, Breath of Love*
2. *Stretching and Relaxation*

3. *Concentration and Awareness*
4. *Gratitude: Healing Images*
5. *Healing the Inner Child*
6. *Forgiveness*
7. *Rainbow Bridge: Harmony of Opposites*

Individual tapes are $10.95 each.
Massachusetts residents please add 5% sales tax.
Send check or money order made out to MIND/BODY HEALTH SCIENCES for the amount of your order plus 20% for postage and handling.
Please allow 3–4 weeks for delivery.

Guilt Is the Teacher, Love Is the Lesson is also available as a book-on-tape through:

Random House Audio Publishing, Inc.
201 East 50th Street
New York, NY 10022

or at your local bookstore.

SERVICES PROVIDED BY JOAN'S ORGANIZATION

MIND/BODY HEALTH SCIENCES also publishes a quarterly newsletter and accepts requests for lectures, workshops, consultations and training by Joan Borysenko, Myrin Borysenko, and other prominent professionals. We provide programs for private, community, religious, health, business, and other organizations.

Please send audiotape orders, program inquiries, and newsletter requests to:

Mind/Body Health Sciences, Inc.
22 Lawson Terrace
Scituate, MA 02066

ON VIDEOCASSETTE

The Power of Myth: Six one-hour interviews of Joseph Campbell with Bill Moyers:

"The Hero's Adventure"
"The Message of the Myth"
"The First Storytellers"
"Sacrifice and Bliss"
"Love and the Goddess"
"Masks of Eternity"

Order from:

Mystic Fire Video
P.O. Box 30969, Dept. VI
New York, NY 10011

PSYCHOSPIRITUAL GROWTH GROUPS

The practice of remembering seems to be easier in community, when groups of people gather together in common cause. Finding such a community to work with is easier in some geographical locations than others, with the exception of twelve-step programs, which are available virtually everywhere. At a workshop, I once commented that it was hard to find group psychospiritual support unless you had an illness or an addiction. I was corrected by several participants who suggested that Alanon, a group for family and friends of alcoholics, was really a group that anyone could join since most everyone's life has in some way been touched by addiction.

Another psychospiritual growth group available across the country to anyone with a personal computer and a modem is an innovative undertaking called Awakening Technology ™. The Awakening Technology Virtual Learning Community is the brainchild and lovechild of Peter and Trudy Johnson-Lenz, who have been doing innovative group work via computer since 1977. They are pioneers in using computers for self-development education and have created a computer-supported learning community of diverse and kindred spirits. They offer a workshop based on *Guilt Is the Teacher, Love Is the Lesson* for people who want to explore the ideas and exercises in this book in the company of others. The community is active, creative, and open—with in-depth personal seminars on different topics, ongoing circles in which people really get to know one another and share, and other on-line events, twenty-four hours a day, seven days a week—on your own home computer. Now that's convenience! If you are interested, write or call Peter and Trudy at:

Awakening Technology℠
695 Fifth Street
Lake Oswego, OR 97034
(503) 635-2615

There's even a money-back guarantee!

EDUCATION AND INFORMATION

The Institute for the Advancement of Health
16 East 53rd Street, Suite 506
New York, NY 10022
(212) 832-8282

The institute for the Advancement of Health (IAH) is for the Mind-Body-Health Field what the American Heart Association is for heart disease or the American Cancer Society is for cancer. IAH has been called the "vanguard of the behavioral medicine movement" by *The New York Times Magazine*. Their excellent journal, *Advances*, provides an authoritative forum for exploring therapies including biofeedback, relaxation, hypnosis, imagery, and stress management. *Advances* is readable and interesting to both the professional and the general public. The Institute separates fact from fiction in an area that is often unscientific. Members receive *Advances* quarterly as well as a newsletter called the *Mind-Body-Health Digest* and special mailings which include information on new research reports, local speakers, and special programs. Individual membership is $39 per year. The Institute was founded in 1983 by Eileen Rockefeller Growald and a distinguished group of psychotherapists, scientists, and laypersons interested in the scientific exploration of the connection between behavior, the mind, the body and health. Please join the Institute for the Advancement of Health now and help support this important effort.

The Institute of Noetic Sciences
475 Gate Five Road, Suite 300
Sausalito, CA 94965
(415) 331-5650
(800) 525-7985 ext. 22-IONS to charge membership on credit card

The institute was founded by astronaut Edgar Mitchell as the result of a profound "holy moment" when he stood on the moon and looked back at the jewel-like planet earth, hanging suspended in the velvet darkness of space. The institute supports research and education on human consciousness. Their goal is "to broaden knowledge of the nature and potentials of mind and consciousness, and to apply that knowledge to the enhancement of the quality of life on the planet." The institute publishes a fascinating quarterly journal, *The Noetic Sciences Review*. They also publish summaries of their excellent research in such areas as psychoneuroimmunology, multiple personality disorder, spontaneous remission, healings at Lourdes, creative altruism and other areas involving mind, body and consciousness. General membership, which includes the *Review* and various other publications, is $35 per year.

AND IN PARTING

A friend gave me a copy of a little poem that she found on a trip to the small town of Arcosanti in Arizona. It lighted Bev's way by awakening her remembrance, and she handed it on to me during a hard time in my life. May it be a light and a blessing to you now, dear friend, in all the steps along your way.

Spirit, *call me son that I may*
seek myself
without tiring

Darkness, *call me brother*
that I may not fear
which I seek

Light, *call me friend*
that I may not be ashamed
by what I see

Death, *call me gently*
that I may enjoy
what I have been.

And Remember

You are not now
Nor have you ever been alone.
From the beginning of time
the human heart
has sought its Source in love.
You are that Source.
You are that love.
Go in peace.

Many blessings.

INDEX

Acceptance, of self, 14, 79, 187–88
Adam and Eve, 144–45, 160–62
Adam, Eve and the Serpent, 144
Addiction, 31, 67
  see also specific addictions
Adult Children of Alcoholics movement, 44, 60, 71
Affect-shame bind, 67
Afflictions, 77, 140–43
  see also specific kinds
Agape, 173
AIDS, 138
Alanon, 44, 71
Alcoholicism, 175–76
  adult children of alcoholics, 43–45, 108
Alcoholics Anonymous, 21, 31, 71, 173
Allison, Ralph, 89
Amends-making, 181
American Journal of Psychiatry, 148
Anger, 9, 48, 71, 205
  fear of, 38
  and forgiveness, 186–87
Anticipation, 1
Antidepressant, 20
Anxiety, 5, 9, 20, 34, 37, 72
  see also Worry
Apologizing, for self, 36–37
Arthritis, 128
Assagioli, Roberto, 61, 87
Assistance, 41–42
Asthma, 11, 55, 198
Auschwitz, 139–40
Awareness. *See* Self-awareness

Bad events, 77, 140–43
Bakker, Jim, 89
Beall, Sandra, 77–78
Becoming Your Own Parent, 44
Being Peace, 135–36
Benson, Herbert, 11, 12, 100, 102, 148
Benson, Peter, 146
Berne, Eric, 60
Bible. *See* New Testament; Old Testament
Biofeedback, 12
Black-and-white thinking, 47–49, 142
Blake, William, 148
Blame
  fixing, 195–97, 200, 201
  God and, 141, 147
  self, 37, 141
Bly, Robert, 62, 63–64, 65
Bodhisattva, 143, 173
Bodymind, 10–14
Boredom, 72
Bradshaw, John, 29, 30–31
Branden, Nathaniel, 45–47
Bridges. *See* Interpersonal bridges: Broken bridges
Bris (circumcision ritual), 105–6
Broken bridges
  false self and, 57, 58–59
  restoring, 72–74, 80
  shame and, 53, 54–57
Bronchitis, 11, 15
Buber, Martin, 188, 189
Buddha and Buddhism, 92, 122, 140, 153, 163, 184, 190
  basic beliefs, 172–73
  bodhisattva, 143, 173
  compassion central to, 173, 176
  metta, 186
  path of insight, 102
  Zen story on forgiveness, 196–97
Byrd, Randolph, 17

Campbell, Joseph, 25, 91–92, 95–96, 157–58, 160–61, 163, 172, 173, 189, 190, 211, 212
Cancer, 152, 153, 215
Caring, 7
  see also Compassion
Casarjian, Robin, 58, 64, 183
Casteneda, Carlos, 187
Catholicism, 19, 106, 123–25, 146, 153–55
Cayce, Edgar, 109
Character disorder, 20
Charity. *See* Compassion
Children, 7, 92
  adult children of alcoholics, 43–45, 60, 71, 108
  emotional pain of, 195–96
  natural state, 1
  shame and trust, 53
  see also Inner child; Natural child
Choice, free, 35
Christ. *See* Jesus Christ
Christianity, 101, 122, 154, 173
  see also Catholicism; Jesus Christ; New Testament; Original Sin
Christian Science, 21
Circumcision, 105–6
City of Joy, 173–74
Clark, Walter Houston, 121
Comforting self, 79–80
Communion, 106
Compassion, 5, 7, 30, 71
  descriptions of, 172–75, 187, 189
  differentiating heaven and hell, 167
  as interpersonal bridge, 96
  see also Forgiveness
Competitiveness, 9
Compliments, 42
Compromise, 194–95
Compulsiveness, 36, 58
Confession, 179–80, 185
Confessions, 144
Conscience, 30
Contentment, 66, 137
Control, 86–87
Coping strategies, 13
Courage, 6, 63
Course in Miracles, A, 19–20, 213
Creative Mythology: The Masks of God, 95
Creativity, 66, 67, 76, 157
Criminals, 30
Crisis, 66
Criticism, 9, 35, 40

David, King, 182, 213
David and Sandy, story of, 197–203
De Chardin, Pierre Teilhard, 194
Defensiveness, 9
Delight, 72
Depression
  causes, 9, 20, 34, 91, 139
  overcoming, 180
Devil, 161, 163–64
Disappointments, 77
Divine Consciousness, 89, 90, 153
Divine nature, 23, 98
Divorce, 55–56, 89
Don Juan, 187
Doors of Perception, The, 148
Dossey, Larry, 15, 16
Drama of the Gifted Child, The, 59
Dreams, 106–13
Dreamwork, 107, 114
Drugs
  abuse, 31, 65
  psychedelic, 148

Eastern philosphy, 148–49, 153, 163. 190
  see also Buddha and Buddhism; Mysticism
Eckhart, Meister, 136, 154
Eddy, Mary Baker, 21
Ego, 104, 134
  death of, 131
Einstein, Albert, 145
Eizik, Isaac, 130, 131
Emmanuel's Book, 25
Empathy, 30
  see also Compassion
Enlightenment, 129–31
Enthusiasm, 66, 91
Envy, 64
Epiphanies, 98
Erhardt, Werner, 60
ESP (extrasensory perception), 119
EST training (Forum), 60
Eve. *See* Adam and Eve
Evil, 161–64
  see also Original sin

False self. *See* Mask
Fainting spells, 11
Fairy tales. *See* Myths
Fanatics, religious, 120
Fatigue, 11, 20
Fault. *See* Blame
Faults, 20, 22
Fear, 20, 71, 134
Feelings, accepting, 14, 79
Female aspect, 130, 198–200
Femme fatale, 56, 58
Fight-or-flight response, 11, 12, 77
Forgiveness, 171–91

compassion and, 172–74
confession and, 179–80
healthy guilt and, 27
Inner Wisdom Exercises, 218–20
and nonjudgmentalness, 6, 189–90
of others, 183–87, 195, 196, 198
of self, 175, 177–83
two sides of, 176–77
For Your Own Good, 59, 65
Forum (EST training), 60
Fox, Matthew, 144, 153–55
Frankl, Viktor, 139
Free choice, 35
Freud, Sigmund, 61, 107–8
Fromm, Erich, 154

Galvani, Luigi, 134
Gender, 198–200
Gibran, Kahlil, 17, 81–82, 112
Ginn, Bob, 78
Giving and receiving, 203–5
Gnostic Gospels, The, 158
Gnosticism, 158–59, 161
God
and blame, 141, 147
and Catholicism, 19, 146
Christian *agape*, 173
female aspect, 130
good and evil, 161–65
and grace, 19, 66, 132, 134, 136
Jewish traditional meditation on, 101
judgment by, 5, 165–67
and mysticism, 120, 123–25, 127–29
nurturing, 155–57, 165
praying to, 181–82, 186, 212–13
and punishment, 138, 141, 142, 144, 148–49, 152
and rituals, 105–6
spiritual conversion, 6, 17, 22, 31, 87, 207
see also Higher Power
Goleman, Daniel, 100, 120
Grace, 19, 66, 105, 131–37, 157, 186, 206
Grail legend, 157–58, 163, 172, 189, 190
Gratitude, 137, 212
Inner Wisdom Exercises, 220–22
Greater Mind/Spirit. *See* Higher Power
Greeley, Andrew, 119, 120, 127
Growth, 205, 209
Guilt
burden of, 3, 86, 197, 198
healing, 13
healthy, 9, 26–27, 29–30
as interface between psychology and religion, 143–45
New Age, 150–53
recovery from, 24
religious, 123–25, 145–47, 138–68
see also Unhealthy guilt

Hanh, Thich Nhat, 135–36, 137
Happiness, 20, 67, 189, 190
Harvard Medical School, 11
Hay, Louise, 150
Headaches, 3, 9–10, 11, 15, 18–19, 65, 198
Heading Toward Omega, 166
Healing, 4, 6, 17, 198
guilt, 13
inner child, 32, 70–82, 146, 202, 216–17
Inner Wisdom Exercises, 72–80, 220–22
soul sickness, 22–25
Healing the Child Within, 32
Healing the Shame That Binds You, 29
Healthy guilt, 9, 26–27, 29–30
Healthy mindedness, 21
Heaven and hell, 167
Heidegger, Martin, 136
Helping, compulsive, 36
Helplessness, 140–42
Helplessness: On Depression, Development and Death, 140
Hero with a Thousand Faces, The, 91–92
Herpes lesions, 123–24
Hesse, Walter, 12
High blood pressure. *see* Hypertension
Higher Power, 6, 17, 31, 87, 207
Hillesum, Etty, 139–40
Hinduism, 122, 130, 149
Hitler, Adolf, 65
Holocaust, 65, 139–40
Holy Grail. *See* Grail legend
Holy Spirit, 130–31
Honoring the Self, 45–47
Hubbard, Celia Thaxter, 214–15
Humility, 187–88
Huxley, Aldous, 61, 121, 148
Hypersensitivity, 9
Hypertension, 3, 9, 11, 15
Hypochondria, 43

Identities, 85–92
self-knowledge, 32–35
"Who am I?" 4, 58, 85–114
see also Mask
Illness, 5
hypochondria, 43
and inner child, 75–78
stress-related, 9–10
see also Medicine, Mind/Body Clinic; specific kinds and symptoms
Imagery exercises, 13–14
Imagination, creative, 76

Imposter syndrome, 38
Inner child, 14, 201
  drama of, 50–69
  guidance, 68–69
  healing, 70–82, 146, 216–17
  and illness, 75–78
  Inner Wisdom Exercises, 72–80, 216–17
  visiting, 74–75
  see also Natural child
Inner Self-Helper, 89–91
Inner Wisdom Exercises, 72–80, 215–22
  forgiveness, 218–20
  gratitude and healing, 220–22
  healing inner child, 216–17
  illness, 75–78
  learning to listen, 78–80
  restoring bridges, 72–74
  visiting inner child, 74–75
Insecurity, 199–200
Insights, 72, 102–3
Insomnia, 11
Institute of Noetic Sciences, 120
Integrated personality, 90, 172, 175
Interpersonal bridges, 52–54, 57, 66, 67, 96
  restoring, 72–74, 80
  see also Broken bridges
Interrupted Life: The Diaries of Etty Hillesum, 1941–1943, An, 139
Intimacy, emotional, 56
Introspection, 3
Intuition, 86–87, 106–13
Ionesco, Eugene, 98, 135
Irritable bowel syndrome, 11
Isolation, 54

James, William, 21–22, 31, 66, 151
Jealousy, 64
Jesus Christ, 23, 58, 132, 140, 153, 155, 159, 162, 173, 176, 189–90
Jews. *See* Judaism and Jews
Joy, 6, 7, 66, 67
Joyce, James, 98
Judaism and Jews
  and mysticism, 100–1, 118, 122, 213
  persecution of, 65, 125, 139–40
  rituals, 105–6
  see also Old Testament
Judgment, by God, 165–67
Judgmentalness. *See* Nonjudgmentalness
Jung, Carl, 21, 22, 24, 59, 61–62, 92, 148–49, 179, 198

Kabat-Zinn, Jon, 11
Kabbala, 101, 118, 122
Kabir, 112, 167–68
Kaufman, Gershen, 30, 31, 53, 67
Keats, John, 6
"Know thyself." *See* Self-knowledge
Kovalski, Stephen, 174
Kübler-Ross, Elisabeth, 51
Kuralt, Charles, 173
Kushner, Harold, 141
Kutz, Ilan, 148–49

LaPierre, Dominique, 173–74
LeBoutillier, Megan, 69
Light Beyond, The, 189
Listening, 78–80
Loneliness, 54
Love, 20, 34
  conditional and unconditional, 51–52, 67, 88
  Divine, 24, 25, 135
  falling in, 192–93
  and grace, 134–37
  human, 192–94
  promises of, 193–94, 200
Lucifer. *See* Devil
Lysis, 66

Malas, 153
Male aspect, 198–200
Mann, Harriett, 74
Man's Search for Meaning, 139
Mantra, 100–1, 212
Many Lives, Many Masters, 142–43
Marriage, 193, 197–98, 199, 200–1
  see also Divorce
Mary Magdalene, 176
Martyr complex, 39
Mask, 65, 67, 68, 88, 93, 172
  false-self models, 57–62
  traits of false and real self, 33
Maslow, Abraham, 97
Maurer, Steve, 22, 104
Medicine, 6
  Era I, 15, 16
  Era II, 16, 20
  Era III, 17, 20
Meditation, 2, 12, 13, 14, 17, 76, 113, 184, 186, 212–13
  basic, 100–4
  Christian, 101
  Kabbalistic tradition, 101
  mantra, 100–1, 212
Meditative Mind, The, 100
Megillat Setarim, 130
Men, 198–200
Merton, Thomas, 113
Metta, 186

Migraine headaches, 9–10, 11, 18–19
Miller, Alice, 59, 65
Milton, John, 167
Mind/Body Clinic, 11, 13, 18, 101, 127, 149, 215
Mind/body techniques, 13, 76
Minding the Body, Mending the Mind, 11, 13, 55, 76, 99, 102, 131, 140, 174, 178
Missildine, Hugh, 74
Mistakes, 9, 181
Mitchell, Edgar, 120
Moody, Raymond, 126, 189
Mother Teresa, 51, 146, 213
Moyers, Bill, 157, 163
Multiple personality, 88–89
"Must" and "should," 40, 199
Mystical experience, 117–18
Mysticism
  Christian, 122, 154
  closet, 119–20
  Eastern, 148–49
  experiencing God, 127
  Kabbala, 101, 118, 122
Myths, 93–96

Nachman, Rabbi, 101, 180, 212–13
Nag Hammadi manuscripts, 158–59
Native Americans, 215
Natural Child, 50, 51, 56–57, 60, 61, 62, 66, 68, 72, 86, 89, 91, 93, 159
  see also Inner child
New Age Journal, 150, 151
New Age movement, 5, 21
  and Eastern mysticism, 149
  guilt, 150–53
  and spiritual pessimism, 147–50
New Testament, 158–59, 189
New Thought movement, 21
"No," fear of saying, 43
Noble Truths, 173
Nonjudgmentalness, 6, 189–90

Old Testament, 112, 143–45, 160, 213
Optimism. *See* Spiritual optimism
Original Blessing, 153–54
Original Sin
  Adam and Eve story, 143–45
  original blessing vew of, 153–54
Orme-Johnson, Rhoda, 98
Overcommitment, 35
Overeaters Anonymous, 71

Pagels, Elaine, 141, 144–45, 151, 158, 161
Pain, 195–96
  see also Affliction; Bad events
Panic attacks, 9, 11, 34
Paradise Lost, 167
Paranoia, 9
Parents
  relationships with, 205–10
  separating from, 80–82
  see also Children
Path of insight, 102–3
Peace, 6, 67, 72
Pennebaker, James, 77–78, 179
Perfectionism, 34, 40–41, 67
Personality
  multiple, 88–89
  well-integrated, 90
Pessimism. *See* Spiritual pessimism
Physical abuse. *See* Punishment
Portrait of the Artist as a Young Man, 98
Positive life. *See* Via Positiva
Power of Myth, The, 96, 157–58, 160–61, 173, 190, 213
Prayer, 181–82, 186, 212–13
  see also Meditation
Present Past, Past Present, 98, 135
Pride, 187–88
Prisoners of Childhood, 59
Problems, 77, 140–43
  see also specific kinds
Prodigal Son, Parable of, 155–57, 164–65, 181
Projection, 64–65
Prophet, The, 81–82
Psychedelic drugs, 148
Psychology, 5, 6
Psychospiritual integration, 90, 172, 175
Psychosynthesis, 61
Punishment, 42, 123–25, 154–55

Quimby, Phineas Parkhurst, 21

Rage, 72
Ramakrishna, 132
Reciprocity, 203–5
Reflection, 183–84
Relationships, 192–210
  giving and receiving, 203–5
  growing up together, 200–3
  growth in, 205
  male and female aspects, 198–200
  with parents, 205–10
Relaxation response, 12, 14
Relaxation Response, The, 102
Religion
  fanaticism, 120
  guilt, 123–25
  and spirituality, 18–19, 22, 120–23

spiritual optimism, 138–68
spiritual pessimism, 145–47
Remembering, touchstones for, 213–15
Remen, Rachel Naomi, 18, 132–33
Repentance, 165
Resentment, 9
Responsibility
in forgiving self, 177–78
in forgiving others, 185
Restore My Soul, 180
Rilke, Rainer Maria, 112, 195
Ring, Kenneth, 126, 166
Rituals, 105–6
Rodegast, Pat, 25

Sabbath, 106
Sadness, 71, 72
St. Augustine, 144–45, 151, 154
St. Francis of Assisi, 190
St. John of Kronstadt, 136–37
Satan. *See* Devil
Satir, Virginia, 59
Saying "no," 43
Scapegoating, 65
Schopenhauer, Arthur, 92
Seductiveness, 67
Seifert, Theodore, 94–95
Self, 48, 66–68, 104
false, 32, 33, 56, 57–62, 157
Higher, 108, 109, 111, 112
Inner Self-Helper, 89–91
learning to experience, 98–99
natural experiences of, 96–98
real, 32, 33
realized, 131, 172
and ritual centering, 105–6
searching for, 24–25, 31, 91–92, 123
true, 32
the Witness, 103
see also Identities; Mask
Self-acceptance, 14, 79, 187–88
Self-awareness, 6, 14, 31, 34, 35, 165, 175, 178
Self-blame, 37, 141
Self-comfort, 79–80
Self-criticism, 9, 35
Self-esteem, 45–47, 146, 188
Selfishness, 41
Self-forgiveness, 175, 177–183
Self-knowledge, 32–35
see also Mask
Self-realization. *See* Enlightenment
Self-respect, 31
Self-righteousness, 65
Seligman, Martin, 140, 141
Separating
from parents, 80–82
task of, 147
Serpent. *See* Adam and Eve
Sex and sexuality, 88–89, 144–45, 205
Shadow, 59, 62–65, 68, 69, 71, 88–89, 93, 108–9, 130–31, 147, 172, 178, 197
Shakti, 130
Shame, 26–49, 144
and broken bridges, 53, 54–57
and conditional love, 67
as false identity, 30–31
identity based on, 35
as innate response, 28–30
and self-esteem, 45–47
and spirituality, 31–32
Shame: The Power of Caring, 30
Sharing, 4, 114
Shekhinah, 130–31
Shiva Sutras, 153
"Should," 40, 199
Shyness, 10
Siegel, Bernie, 132
Sins, 42, 138, 146, 164–65
see also Original Sin; Punishment
Skinner, B. F., 154, 155
Smith, Huston, 160
Snow White, 93–95
Snow White: Life Almost Lost, 94–95
Solomon, King, 182
Song of Solomon, 112
Song of Songs, 112
Soul, 24, 58, 67
dark night of, 129–31
and spirit, 14–17
Soul sickness, 31, 58
healing, 22–25
as unhealthy guilt, 19–22
Spectrum of Consciousness, 151
Spilka, Bernard, 146
Spirit, 24, 51, 66, 89
see also Higher Power; Self
Spiritual exercises, 211–22
Inner Wisdom, 215–22
practices of remembering, 212–13
touchstones for remembering, 213–15
Spirituality
and religion, 18–19, 22, 120–23
and shame, 31–32
Spiritual longing, 31
Spiritual optimism, 5, 18
and religious guilt, 138–68
traditions of, 153–55
transformations, 159–68
Spiritual pessimism, 5, 18, 19
and New Age philosophy, 147–50
and religious guilt, 145–47
shadow of, 147

Spiritual plane, 96
Spiritual revision, 115–37
  closet mystics, 119–20
  enlightenment, 129–31
  grace, 131–37
  looking within, 116–19
  religion or spirituality, 120–23
  religious guilt, 123–25
Spiritual search, 4
Spiritual sphere of knowledge, 5
Stanton, Judith, 25
Stress, 3, 9–10, 11
Subpersonalities, 87
Suffering, 6
  see also Afflictions; Bad events
Swaggart, Jimmy, 89

Tagore, Rabindranath, 112, 113
Tarot cards, 110–11
Taylor, Jeremy, 107, 109–10, 111–12, 114
Temporal realm, 4, 96
Tennyson, Alfred Lord, 112
Touchstones, 213–15
Tower Dream, 110–11
Transactional analysis, 60
Traumas, 77, 78
Travers, P. L. 171–72, 175, 211
Troubles, 77, 140–43
  see also specific kinds
Trust, 53, 129
Truth, 63

Ulcers, 11, 183
Unhealthy guilt, 1, 3, 4, 9, 22, 26, 27, 34, 86, 88
  adult children of alcoholics, 43–45
  expressions of, 35–43
  religion-inspired, 123–25
  and shame, 26–49
  and soul sickness, 19–22

Varieties of Religious Experience, The, 21
Via Positiva, 154–55
Victims, 133
Viorst, Judith, 193
Visions, 165–66

Wallace, R. Keith, 12
Ware, Archimandrite Kallistos, 97
Weiss, Brian, 142–43, 153
When Bad Things Happen to Good People, 141
Whitfield, Charles, 32, 44
Whitman, Walt, 112
"Who am I?" 4, 58, 85–114
  dreams and intuition, 106–13
  meditation, 100–4
  myths, 93–96
  ritual centering, 105–6
Wholey, Dennis, 44
Wilber, Ken, 151
Wilber, Treya Killam, 151
Wilder, Thornton, 4
Wisdom, 6, 66, 67, 72, 160
  psychological-spiritual union, 157–59
Witnessing, 103, 113
Women
  female aspects, 130, 198–200
  femme fatale, 56, 58
Workaholism, 57, 108
Worry, 35–36, 37–38, 39–40, 42, 43
Worthiness, 7, 23

Yoga, 99
You Can Heal Your Life, 150

Zen, 196–97